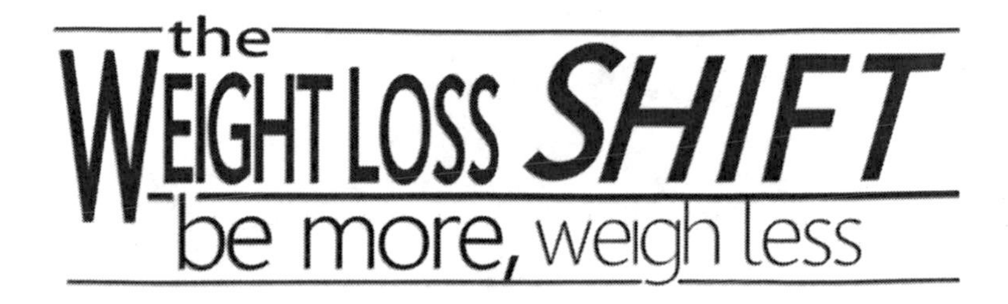

By Michelle Hastie

Absolute Love Publishing

Absolute Love Publishing

The Weight Loss Shift: Be More, Weigh Less
By Michelle Hastie

Published by Absolute Love Publishing

USA

Edited by Sarah Hackley

Cover design by Brandi Lyons

United States of America

The Weight Loss Shift:

Be More, Weigh Less

By Michelle Hastie

Dear readers,

Join me for your weight loss shift!

I'd love to invite you to join an incredible group of ex-dieters who are learning to shift their weight and finally live in their ideal bodies for good. Here's how:

1. Sign up to get free book bonuses, inspiring blogs, updates, and specials just for my tribe at http://totalbodyhealthsolutions.com/weightlossshiftbonus/

2. If you enjoyed this book, please share it with loved ones and add a review on Amazon, Barnes and Noble, Goodreads, or any other book review site!

Sincerely, Michelle

I dedicate this book to the love of my life, the man who pushed me to start a business, supported me in the times I failed miserably, and will continue to stand by me and watch my dreams come true. I love you, Nicklas.

Contents

How to Use This Book

Most weight loss books give you a strict list of rules to follow and foods to eat. They tell you what to do, and you do it – to the best of your ability – in the hopes that you will then have the results you desire. This book is different.

Instead of immediately telling you **what to do**, this book first tells you **how to be**. It explains the distinction and gives you an actionable plan for how to make the jump from who you are to who you want to be. Only then does it offer advice on what to do.

To get the most out of this book, you must read it in order.

For reasons I explain in the first chapter, "being" is much more relevant to your weight loss goals than "doing." If you skip ahead to the "doing" section without first reading, understanding, and implementing the homework exercises in the "being" section, you will not achieve the results you want.

This will be difficult. We are naturally inclined to want to move right into what we need to do to get results, and this inclination is rewarded in our society. Often we are thought of as lazy if we are not constantly in doing mode, and we are praised when we work to achieve our goals. But, sometimes, we make more progress toward those goals when we are still than when we are moving.

For example, while many people might say that lying in bed watching movies all day is a complete waste of time, I find it rejuvenating. Taking a full day to recuperate in this way is what enables me to be so productive on other days. It's what gives me the energy and motivation to take the time to cook healthy meals and go to yoga. Without days like this, many of our daily activities turn into stress-ridden obligations.

If you truly want to lose weight long term and achieve your ideal body, you are going to have to trust in the being-instead-of-doing process. You are going to have to dig deep under the surface to find real answers about who you are and who you want to be. You will be asked to throw out old belief systems that are no longer serving you and to admit that you are ready for new answers and systems that resonate more fully with your ideal self.

You must be open to these new thoughts. Open to changing your beliefs about how your body works. Open to throwing away ideas you have carried around on your back for years and, instead, claiming new thought patterns.

This is not necessarily easy.

It's possible each of the principles in this book will shake your model of the world and compete with the knowledge you have been given about weight loss up to this point. Some things I say may sound ludicrous or too good to be true. But, I will be sure to give evidence for every truth principle I state, helping calm your inner skeptic and enabling you to put these principles to use.

The rest is on you. It's on you, on you, on you. If you can open yourself up to this book and the process described within these pages, you will achieve the results you desire.

I have been living in my ideal body effortlessly since I mastered this information. And, so can you. In fact, you don't have to stop there. All the principles I discuss here can be used to find love, launch a new career, or accomplish anything else your heart desires.

It's fairly simple: You read this book, you open your mind to new truths that enable you to have a life you love, and you make changes immediately.

No more "the diet starts Monday." Once the weight loss process isn't filled with deprivation, force, starvation, pain, and punishment, you will not want to push it back to Monday. You'll want to start today – right now!

So start. Start today, right now. But, start at the beginning of this book, and work your way through. As you read through the pages, take your time. Read them over and over again. Work through the questions that are posed to you in each section. Journal when resistance comes up. Notice when your mind tries to tell you that you can't do it, and then correct that lie. Stay present with the words, and honor the parts that sing to you. Discard the ones that don't.

Remember to stay true to you, your highest self, not your fear-based self that is terrified to change. Feel the fears and keep moving forward anyway with courage and strength. Invite other like-minded women and men to read as well and discuss weekly in groups honoring each others' fears and dreams.

And, if you really want to get the most out of this book, find creative ways to interpret, solidify, and embody the words in ways that are fun and inspiring. The more color the better! Use crayons, colored pencils, paints, and collages to allow this information to sink in even deeper. If you make this book a study, your life will absolutely change, just as soon as you are ready and open to "be."

The Truth

I'm guessing you are sick and tired of hearing the same b.s. about how to lose weight. You hear it on TV, on the radio, and at the gym. You read about it in newspapers and magazines. And, everyone, from your mom and your best friend to your hairstylist and your mail carrier, has some new tip he or she just **has** to share:

"All you need to do is eat less and move more."

"What's wrong with you, don't you have any willpower?"

"Get your butt off the couch and move!"

"Just work out two times a day."

"Don't you want it bad enough?"

But you've tried it, all of it, and none of it works. No matter what you do, what crazy fad diet you try or intense workout plan you follow, the weight doesn't come off, at least not long term. Eventually, you get disheartened, beating yourself up for not being able to cut out carbs completely or for not getting up every morning at 6 to hit the gym. So, you start looking again, swearing that next time you'll be better, work harder, eat less, do more, that the next weight loss "fix" is right around the corner.

But, guess what? You're not the problem. The problem is with what you're being told, because every bit of it is wrong.

Let me repeat that: **Every bit of conventional advice you've been given about how to lose weight and keep it off is wrong.**

"How can that be?" I hear you asking. How can everyone, from the so-called "weight loss" experts on TV and in magazines to your best friend who just lost five pounds on the latest fad diet, be wrong?

Most people in your life – the experts, your family, the nail salon owner – they all mean well. They want to see you happy and feeling good in your body. They want you to be healthy. But, the truth is, they don't know how to get you there.

They think they know, but they have no idea, because **they are all tackling weight loss from the wrong starting point.**

Why the So-Called "Experts" are Wrong

There are two main reasons conventional weight loss advice doesn't work. The first is built on a flawed understanding of how our bodies work and a false assumption that we're all the same. The second concerns a focus on temporary instead of long-term results.

Standard weight loss advice is built on the assumption that there is a cookie-cutter formula that you can follow the steps of and lose weight. As if we are all exactly the same and anyone can simply follow the "expert's" formula and *Voila*! have the exact same results.

And honestly, that is what you want to believe, too. Most of us want someone to dish out a cookie-cutter formula that tells us what to do from the minute we wake up to the minute we go to sleep, one that guarantees we will live the life the thin, happy "experts" live. But, the down and dirty truth is there is no such thing as a cookie-cutter formula, because we're all different.

I could put three of my weight loss coaching clients in one room for 30 days and have them all do the exact same thing at the exact same time, and all their results would be different. This is the reality. The more you allow yourself to embrace this truth, the more empowered you will be moving forward. Without complete honesty in any personal development or self-growth work, your results always will be temporary at best, and temporary results are what you want to avoid. This is the second way in which conventional advice goes wrong.

Standard weight loss advice is all about getting the weight off – very rarely does it realistically concern itself with *keeping* it off. Consider a friend who has been raving for the past 30 days about the new "revolutionary" diet that has completely changed her life. You notice she's looking thinner so you figure it must be working. Then, you go to her house for dinner.

There are no carbs on her plate, and her portions are much smaller than they have been in the past, but those aren't the only changes you see. She's devouring her food, scarfing it down so quickly it's difficult to believe she even registers the taste. She also appears to be about one second away from picking up her plate and licking it clean. And, she's analyzing the meal the entire time, reciting how many calories are in each part of the meal and how much she will be working out the next day to ensure she doesn't gain weight.

Can that possibly be sustainable? Not likely. Even if it were, is that how you want to live? Watching what you eat and eating without enjoyment for the rest of your life? I hope not!

There is a reason all diets fail and/or yield only temporary results. It's because they are bloody awful. They aren't considering how the advice or program influences your life on a long-term basis, and they do not align with your highest and most authentic self.

Thankfully, there is another way.

There is a way to lose weight, keep it off, and live your life happily, without becoming obsessed with counting calories and working out.

There is a way to be thin, love your body, and live completely free of worry about your weight.

There are people, right now, who can say in complete honesty that they don't fear weight gain. That they aren't worried about eating sweets, carbs, or fat. That they don't feel guilty if they miss a day at the gym.

I'm one of these people.

You can be one of these people, too.

And, you don't have to get up and work out at 5 a.m. every day or cut out your favorite foods or become a slave to your scale to get there. You don't have to follow any of the standard weight loss advice. Instead, all you have to do is *change who you are being.*

This has nothing to do with what you eat or how much you move. It's about the programs you run in your mind and how they dictate the results in your life.

This idea may seem strange at first, but think about this: In following conventional weight loss advice, you've been "doing" a bunch of things in order to "have" the body that you believe will cause you to "be" someone who lives an incredible life. However, if you're honest with yourself, you'll realize you aren't really looking for a smaller and/or lighter body; you are searching for fulfillment, happiness, and/or love for yourself. And, you've been expecting these results, the "being" someone with an incredible life, to come from the "doing."

You think if you lose weight and change your appearance, you will have these things. But, that isn't the case. When you skip the "being" step, you'll never get the results you want, and the results you find fulfilling, at least not in the long term.

To get an incredible life, you must first "be" the person who lives an incredible life.

If you want a life free of restrictions, deprivation, starvation, and limitations, you must first be a person who lives without limitations, without restrictions. Someone who doesn't starve or deprive yourself of the things you need and desire. You must feel the feelings, and understand the decisions, of someone who is actually living the life you desire. Then, you will automatically start "doing" things the way this other person does them. **And, you'll get what you want – fulfillment, happiness, and love for yourself – right away, not once the weight comes off**.

So stop listening to those know-it-alls who say you have to follow *their* rules. You don't need others' rules.

When you change who you are being, you start approaching life from a place of self-love and self-care. You start doing more things for yourself. You begin giving yourself the things you truly want and need. And, then, your whole life changes.

That person you were, you know the person who would beat herself up for eating that cupcake (or two) at the party last week? She's gone.

The person who would agonize over the fact that he skipped the gym three times last week? He's gone.

And that person you used to envy, the one who somehow stops when she is full, craves a great workout, or is annoyed when he can't get to his yoga class ... that's you.

Suddenly, the overeating goes away, the binge eating subsides, your desire for movement aligns itself with your true needs, and the weight falls off.

So, now, how do you get there?

You learn the truth.

What is Our Truth?

I talk to people every day who believe they have gained weight because of overconsumption and under movement. I also talk to people who are thin, who believe that all people with excess weight are lazy and don't have willpower. The truth is: Neither one of these statements is true because they are both based on the same flawed belief, the same flawed assumption.

You have heard of "calories in versus calories out." According to conventional advice, it is the #1 method to losing weight. In fact, in many circles, including in the gym I first started working in, it is the ONLY way to lose weight. But, guess what? **It doesn't work, and believing in it actually sabotages your weight loss efforts.** Let me explain.

The calorie argument is derived from one of the "Laws of Thermodynamics," but as with most scientific laws, these laws are describing a perfect, *idealized* process, in this case an idealized thermodynamic process in an idealized thermodynamic system.

For the calories in versus calories out "law" to be foolproof, our bodies would have to be exactly the same. We all would have to experience the exact same amount of stress and emotions. We would all need to have the exact same hormones and genetics. We don't have any of these things so these variances in the way we each, individually, "consume life" throw this law out the window.

How else could we know the horror (as I sure do) of cutting calories to 1200 per day, working out five days a week at high intensity, and still climbing on the scale after 30 days to see an increase?

Our bodies, as far as theoretical science is concerned, are not ideal systems. They are unique and wonderful systems that need different things, desire different things, and react to different things. But, it isn't easy to throw this idea away.

Even I, who once worked out two times a day, seven days a week, for a year-and-a-half, resisted the idea that this so-called law could be bogus, even when I got heavier and heavier as the days went by. But, despite the resistance you'll feel initially, it is imperative to your success in your body and weight that you divorce yourself from this method of weight loss completely. Why? Because following the rule of calories in versus calories out means you're making your meal decisions and your life decisions based on a number written on a menu or on a workout program or on the Internet, instead of based on what your body needs and desires.

This is completely backwards.

Counting calories can work, but never long term. You can trick your body into losing weight on the calories in versus calories out system, but only temporarily. Your body will always catch up to you because you're a person, not an idealized "system."

You get stressed, and then you process food differently than someone who isn't stressed. Your basal metabolic rate (the number of calories that you supposedly burn just by living) changes because you've been dieting or because you put on muscle. You drink too little water one day and your organs work less efficiently. There are countless ways in which your body expresses its complexity and uniqueness and, therefore, drifts further away from the idealized system the laws of thermodynamics are meant to explain.

This is why someone can barely eat and still gain weight, and why another person can eat everything on his or her plate and yours and still be thin. The truth is, I followed the rule of calories in and calories out, and it didn't work for me. I had clients who followed this "scientific law," and it didn't work for them, either.

You may want to write the differences off to "good genes" or willpower or intensity, but that's incorrect. If you want to lose weight long term, and get the life you want, you will have to accept the fact that weight loss isn't a simple adjustment of food and/or exercise. You must accept that it's complex and intuitive, ever changing and transformative. And, that acceptance will lead you through the inspiring, enlightening, and enjoyable experience of changing who you are *being* into the awesome reality of living your best life as a lighter, and healthier, you.

Be

Some of you are going to want to breeze through this section, or simply skip it altogether. You will think: "Yeah, yeah this might be important for some people, but I just need to be told what to do." If that is you, you **must** read this chapter, preferably more than once, before you move on to the "doing" part. Why? Because you cannot weigh less by doing more. To get what you want, you must become the person who has the body and life you want.

Changing your identity – creating the you who lives your ideal life – is the entire focus of this section. But, before you can get to work changing who you're being, you must first be honest about who you are right now. And, that takes understanding the difference between someone who is living with excess weight they don't want and someone who is living in his or her ideal body.

Living from an Overweight Consciousness

Those of you who are operating your life from overweight consciousness (which, by the way, doesn't mean you have to be overweight) have a general belief in limitations in your body and life. In other words, you have bought into the idea that your body needs to be manipulated or changed externally to have the internal world you desire. There is a lack of trust in the body and therefore you rely on a lot of external help, which ultimately doesn't allow the body to do what it does best, naturally.

You have feelings of being lost, scared, and unsure of what to do next. You maintain a constant obsession over pounds, inches, calories, and everything weight related, which is why even thin people can operate from this space.

There is usually a controlling nature and a fear to simply let go and trust that anything is possible. You desire to control either everything that goes in the body or everything that goes out of the body in order to feel safe.

You most likely experience deprivation, especially around food, which creates a negative relationship with food, exercise, and your body. You also feel heavy, and everything feels difficult.

There is an overall lack of awareness and communication with your body, which doesn't allow you to listen to your body's symptoms and messages. If asked, "What does your body want right now?" you often will feel blocked or too confused to answer. In short, your life revolves around your constant worry about your weight.

Operating from an Ideal Weight Consciousness

Those of you operating from ideal weight consciousness have an absolute trust in your body. This allows you to do whatever your inner voice says, whether it is asking for a salad and a run or pasta and a nap.

You have high self-worth and self-love. You allow yourself to feel your emotions, even when they are unpleasant, as opposed to stuffing them down and using avoidance. You have a healthy relationship with food, exercise, and your body, and everything feels light and easy.

You operate from a place of abundance around food, and nothing is off limits or lacking. You are living in the deepest, most authentic version of yourself, which helps you create an incredible life of health, wealth, and transformation.

Starting the Transformation

Which consciousness are you operating in right now? Be honest about where you are, without judgment. If you are in "overweight consciousness," don't worry! This entire section will re-educate you so that you can align with your truth and "be" in your ideal body. Remember: There is only one way to transform, and that's to start from where you are.

Being the Person Who Gets Results

To get the body and life you want, you must become the person who effortlessly gets and maintains the results you desire. To do that, you must recognize several important truths about how your thoughts, emotions, stressors, and desires affect your results.

Your Subconscious Programming Determines Your Weight

I am sure you have said things like, "Oh that's just my subconscious talking," or "Subconsciously I must have known you were calling." We talk about our subconscious mind with competence and understanding, but we don't truly understand what it is, what it does, and how it works.

The subconscious mind:

Stores and organizes memories

Is the domain of the emotions
Represses memories with unresolved negative emotions
Presents repressed memories for resolution
May keep the repressed emotions repressed for protection
Runs the body
Preserves the body
Is a highly moral being
Enjoys serving and needs clear orders to follow
Controls and maintains all perceptions
Generates, stores, distributes, and transmits energy
Maintains instincts and generates habits
Needs repetition until a habit is installed
Is programmed to continually seek more and more
Functions best as a whole integrated unit
Is symbolic
Takes everything personally
Works on the principle of least effort
Does not process negatives

Your subconscious mind stores everything that happens to you in life: every belief, value, event, and sensory experience. It runs constantly, whether you are awake or asleep.

Your subconscious mind is what allows you to drive your car without thinking about every little thing, and to block out unnecessary sounds and sights so you don't go into sensory overload. It also processes information so you don't consciously have to think about everything all at once. Most importantly, its role in your life varies, depending on your age.

From the ages of 0-7, you are considered to be a walking unconscious mind. This means that everything happening around you and said to you simply goes into your mind and is stored, without your ability to decide if you want to believe it or not.

After the age of 7, your unconscious mind fades into the background as you become able to decide whether you want to believe something or call it absurd.

For example, you can tell small children, “The sky is purple,” and they will begin to contemplate how this is possible or ask more questions to clarify why they are seeing something different. They are completely open to the idea that the sky may, in fact, be purple.

If you tell an adult, “The sky is purple,” he or she will simply write you off and move on with the day.

This means, that as adults, most of us are operating our lives based on beliefs that were created in our minds, without our conscious thoughts, from the age of 0-7.

Why is it important to acknowledge this? Because we have to be honest about why we think what we think and do what we do. Often, it has nothing to do with our decisions as adults.

For example, if a girl was raised in a home in which her mom was obsessed with her body and losing weight, then that girl has been conditioned to believe being obsessed with her weight is a part of normal, everyday life. It doesn't matter if she wants to believe that, her exposure to it at such a young age means she didn't have a choice.

Now, as an adult, she likely either mimics the experience of her mother and struggles with her weight on a daily basis or she is so terrified of living the way her mother lived that she finds herself obsessed with staying thin.

I'm not suggesting we blame our parents for our troubles. I'm simply pointing out that our experiences in early childhood shape who we become as adults. We must acknowledge this in order to understand our current thoughts, beliefs, and patterns.

Ask yourself:

Who taught you that you needed to lose weight?

When did you decide that excess weight is unhealthy? Or unappealing? Or ugly?

Where did you pick up the pattern to control everything?

When did you begin to always expect the worst?

You might not be able to specifically pin down the answers to these questions, but I can venture a guess that it is all related to your childhood experiences at a very young age.

This is vital because if you were given the belief at a young age that losing weight is hard ...

Or that you are fat ...

Or that you are not meant to be thin ...

Or that thin people are bad ...

Then, you can keep saying you want to lose weight, but it won't happen because your subconscious mind digs through your beliefs before acting, looking for discrepancies between what you say and what you think.

Your thoughts and beliefs are immensely powerful. They create who you are, what you do, and what you have. If you can begin to separate out the beliefs that are no longer serving you, especially those that aren't even your beliefs to begin with, you will become successful and achieve the things you want.

You easily will let go of the ideas that are holding you back, and begin to choose beliefs that motivate you and bring you closer to your ideal self. You will begin substituting negative thoughts, such as "I'm not acceptable as I am" and "I must diet to lose weight and be loved," with positive ones, such as "Accepting myself means being happy at any weight" and "Loving myself is a better way to achieve the results I desire."

Not only will this make you feel better and hasten your weight loss journey, but it also will make you more powerful. By replacing your old thoughts with new thoughts that better serve you, you will be bringing your thoughts and beliefs into alignment with where you want to go, as opposed to where you were or have been. This alignment will then strengthen the attraction between you and the things you want, bringing you into contact with the life and body you desire.

To get there, however, you have to let go, let go of your need for control and allow your subconscious mind to take over. This last part is important. You want your subconscious mind in charge, because **it is the only way to get the results you want**.

Oftentimes I hear people say that they just want to be able to eat food, move their bodies, live their lives, and achieve their ideal weight. They wonder if this is too much to ask. To me this is their way of saying they want weight loss to be automatic. They don't want to have to think about it so much, they just want it to happen in the background while they focus on living their life. To which I respond, "Why would it be any other way?"

You have a purpose. You were born for a reason. And unless you feel your purpose is to lose weight, it makes sense that you don't want your focus and attention to be on forcing your way to a lighter you. Unfortunately, we have been trained from a young age to "keep our eyes on the prize," and work our way to the finish line, so letting go and allowing our subconscious minds to take over is difficult. Remember though, this journey isn't about doing more. It is about *being more*.

In reality, you will release the weight so much faster if you can take your focus off of weight loss and turn it toward living an incredible life.

To do this, you must begin changing who you are being (your identity) by changing your thoughts and beliefs.

Your identity is described in those statements you make that start with "I am." If you are saying to yourself "I am overweight" or "I am fat," your values and beliefs will align with that identity. You will be what you say you are. To change who that is, you must begin describing yourself as you want to be. You must begin describing yourself as someone living in his or her ideal body would. *However, these statements must be something you can believe.*

You can't just walk around saying, "I am thin," if you aren't or do not believe you are. Your emotions and feelings would not be in alignment with that, and you would feel as though you were telling yourself a big, fat lie. Every time you looked in the mirror you would prove your statements to be untrue, and this would take you further from your goals.

Instead, you must find and adopt "I am" statements that you can believe, such as:

"I love myself at this weight."

"I am lovable."

"It's wonderful that I can live in my ideal body."

"I am valuable at every weight."

TIP: A positive "I am" statement about absolutely anything is better than any negative "I am" statement about your weight.

Homework Assignment #1
Finding the True Version of You

Your first homework assignment is to write down all the parts of you that aren't really you, the parts that are other people's voices living rent-free in your head. Then write down all the parts that are you and the parts of who you want to become. This will help you identify where you are now and where you want to be. It also will get you started on the path to replacing your negative "I am" statements with positive ones.

For example:

I have been operating by the following beliefs:

I am fat.
I am unworthy.
I am not athletic.

I know the following to be absolutely true:

I am human.
I am a spiritual being living in a physical body.
I am kind and loving.
I am constantly growing.
I am willing to let go of all the beliefs that are no longer serving me.

I am becoming:

A person who spends my time enjoying the activities that matter most to me.
Someone with unbounded energy and enthusiasm.
A person who is happy with his/her body.
A person who is happy with his/her life.

Setting the Stage

Digging deep into who you've been, who you are, and who you want to be can be a very emotional process. Give yourself the proper time and space to do this by:

Stepping out in nature or settling into a room in your home that makes you feel nurtured and protected.

Grabbing a cup of chamomile tea and some fuzzy slippers or whatever brings you comfort.

Playing some light music in the background.

Buying a beautiful journal and pen and designating them just for these types of activities.

Once you've set the stage, surround yourself with anything and everything that makes you feel safe. Then, dive in to this exercise and imagine your way to the new you!

Your Emotions Are Here to Teach You Lessons, Not Make You Fat

We've all blamed our weight gain on emotional eating. The truth, however, is that emotional eating is not the exclusive domain of the overweight. It's universal.

We all eat foods for emotional reasons. We reach for one food because it reminds us of our childhoods, for another because it makes us feel safe or secure. We stock up on our favorite feel-good foods when we're sick or trying to mend a broken heart. We eat when we're sad and when we're happy and in celebration.

If emotional eating is such a normal part of our lives, the question becomes: Why do some people gain weight when they do it while others don't?

The difference is not in what or when we eat. It's in **how** we eat, and how we deal with the underlying emotions causing us to eat.

Both thin and overweight people may use a pint of ice cream to deal with a break up, but they do so very differently. While overweight people may dig into the ice cream when they're already full, thin people will wait until they are hungry to eat it. Then, unlike overweight people who often rush through the treat, berating themselves for their lack of willpower, thin people will be present with the food as they eat, taking their time with it and savoring each feel-good bite. Finally, when it's done, it's done, no follow-up serving of guilt or judgment.

When we eat out of emotional hunger without any physical hunger, we introduce negativity into the experience from the very beginning. Right away, we acknowledge that we are ignoring our body, which we don't like, and then we proceed to make ourselves physically uncomfortable. Our discomfort causes us to withdraw from the eating experience, making it largely unconscious. When we do this, we also withdraw from our emotions. Then, because we haven't been present, we do not get the feel-good experience we were expecting, and we look for more. Suddenly, the pint of ice cream turns into a pint-and-a-half of ice cream, plus a bag of chips and ten cookies.

Once we snap out of our emotional binge, we feel overly full, guilty, and judgmental of ourselves. In the end, we feel worse than we did when we started. Instead of feeling like we've taken care of ourselves, we feel betrayed. Instead of loved, we feel pained. And, we are still left to deal with the emotion that caused us to want the ice cream in the first place, which means the entire process inevitably will repeat itself, unless we figure out how to break the cycle. Learning how to effectively handle painful emotions is one way to do this.

Oftentimes when we feel anger, sadness, guilt, fear, doubt, or any other emotion we don't enjoy feeling, our first inclination is to stop feeling it immediately. This inclination, however, often backfires, because it violates two important emotional truths:

1. Allowing ourselves to feel our unenjoyable emotions drastically reduces their intensity.

2. The less we resist unenjoyable emotions, the faster they subside and we can move on.

By attempting to flee from our emotions, we are only postponing the inevitable moment when we will be required to deal with them. We would be better served if we took the time to understand them.

Whatever unenjoyable emotion you may be feeling, consider why you are feeling it. If it is an emotion you continue to feel over and over, like fear, consider what lessons the emotion may have to teach you.

If you can identify what you are meant to learn from fear, you won't need to feel it so often. If you know why you have doubt, your body won't need to keep sending you the message. Remember: The subconscious mind communicates to us through pictures, sounds, and feelings. Your conscious mind's job is to figure out those communications and learn from them.

When you feel like eating and you know you are not physically hungry, ask yourself what you really need in that moment. Be open and honor your body and mind and what it requires of you. Once you learn to face your emotions head-on, you'll stop covering them up with food, and the binges will stop.

Homework Assignment #2
Releasing Fears and Embracing Feelings

Write down the reasons you may be fleeing from your emotions. What are you afraid will happen if you feel them completely? Are you afraid of being like one of your parents or of being too sensitive? What is the part of you that is disallowing you to dive into your emotions, feel them, and heal from them? What is so painful?

Once you have identified your fears, follow each one up with a truth statement. Remind yourself that no emotion lasts forever, and that by fully feeling it you will be able to release it that much sooner. Tell yourself that you are practicing self-care by facing the reality of your feelings.

When you are able to identify what you are afraid of much of the fear will subside, and you will be able to learn the lessons you need to learn and move on (without the pint of ice cream).

For Example:

Fear: I am afraid that if I allow myself to feel anxiety without trying to get it to go away it will stay forever. If it stays forever, I will never be able to take a full breath, and I want to be able to breathe fully.

Truth Statement: I intellectually know that anxiety won't be in my life forever, and I welcome it into my life for the short duration it needs to be here. I acknowledge that allowing myself to feel anxiety enables me to release it that much sooner.

Setting the Stage

Feeling your emotions can take some practice, and it can be hard work, especially if you have been pushing them away for a long time. Start by noticing the subtle changes in your body when you feel good versus when you feel bad. When you feel bad, where do you feel it in your body? When you feel good, where do you feel it in your body? Notice how your muscles feel, what your face is doing, what your breath sounds like, and how you hold your body in each instance.

Emotions need to be expressed. If you have been pushing them away for a long time, they will want to come up over and over and over for a little while. Allow this to happen. Allow them to have a voice so you can move on and let them out of your body.

Your Internal Stressors Create Your External World

Are you aware of what stress does to you?

In addition to affecting every cell in your body, it causes sleeplessness, mood swings, and low energy. It also wreaks havoc on your weight loss goals by causing your body to store fat and burn muscle and by negatively impacting your digestion and metabolism.

This means that if you are under high-level or even low-level chronic stress it doesn't matter what you do in terms of weight loss efforts, you will have difficulty removing your weight.

If you're operating from a place of stress, all the health magazine tricks in the world won't help you speed up your metabolism and lose weight. You can eat breakfast and six small meals a day, you can drink caffeine and green tea, take diet pills, restrict certain foods – none of it will matter. The only thing that matters is the stress. Reduce or eliminate the stress, and you'll speed up your metabolism and begin to lose weight. But how?

You slow down, and you relax.

How you do this, however, will depend on whether your chronic stress is caused by external or internal factors.

We are all very familiar with external stress, which could be relationship stress, money stress, or work stress. Internal stress is what you create in your own mind, just for you. It's like a little gift you bought yourself, but one you want to return right away.

It's that tape that plays over and over in your head every day. If you have thoughts like, "I look fat," "I'm unlovable," "I am a failure," "I am not worth it," then you are flooding your body with the same amount of stress hormones as you would be if you were being chased by a lion (a potent external stressor).

Just like external stress, internal stress often comes from fear. The difference, however, is that with internal stress the stressor isn't real – you have created it.

Your heart may be pounding. Your breath may be coming in shallow gasps. You may be panicked, but the stress and the fear aren't real. You have created them. *And, because you created them, you also can destroy them.* The trick is finding a way to deal with the stress and the fear effectively.

How do you handle stressful situations? Do you have problem solving strategies or do you ignore the stress, hoping it will go away?

When I am stressed, I often stop everything I am doing to meditate or go be in nature. This gives me the chance to decompress and let my fears and anxieties go.

For those of you who are thinking it would be nice to drop everything and go to the beach BUT you have other, more important, things to do, you are wrong. Trying to power through your stress will never work. Think about how your mind works. If it's full of chatter, you cannot make clear intelligent decisions.

You have to stop and get rid of stress if you want to move forward efficiently. This might mean going to the gym or taking a nap or something else altogether. The trick is finding what works for you. Do you need stillness or movement? Do you need to be alone or does it help to be around others? Do you need time off? Need to spend time being creative? What does your body need? Discover what serves you in your life, and use it.

Homework Assignment #3
Total Thoughts Assessment

Answer the following questions:

1. What are the external stressors affecting you right now?
2. What are the internal stressors affecting you right now?
3. How “real” are those stressors?
4. What are your coping strategies?
5. How well are those strategies working for you?
6. Are there things you could be doing that would work better?
7. What do you really need to decompress and release the stress in your life?

For Example:

1. I have a demanding boss I feel I can’t please, and a friend who is overly needy.
2. I allow the process of losing weight to be a large burden and stressor in my life. I feel like I have to be perfect, and it’s hard. I stress over my body every time I look in the mirror.
3. My boss is demanding, but she also praises me for a job well done, so I probably don’t need to feel stress that I am inadequate. My friend is needy, but maybe I just haven’t said “no” enough. Stressing over my weight is something I don’t need in my life, but I’m not sure how to fix it – yet.
4. I cope by eating and vegging out in front of the TV.
5. Not well, especially when it comes to my weight. My strategies only make me feel worse.

6. I could practice yoga or take a long walk or a bubble bath. I could call a friend and chat.
7. I could learn to say “no” when people ask more of me than I want to give, and I could learn to approach my weight and my body with love instead of criticism.

Setting the Stage

This exercise takes a great deal of honesty. Remember: It’s not about blame or guilt. Acknowledge that you have been doing the best you could with the tools you had up to this point and honor your journey. Then, commit to paying attention to what your body truly needs and letting the rest of it go.

You Have to See Where You Are Going Before You Can Get There

Likely there have been plenty of times when you've said to yourself: "This is it! I am losing the weight! This time is for real!" You then ride out your new sense of excitement and you are unstoppable: Staying in your calorie range isn't so hard. Going to the gym isn't such a big deal, and you go on your merry way thinking, "This is it, I finally figured it out!"

Then something happens, and you lose motivation. The scale goes up or doesn't change after working out hard seven days in a row and eating perfectly. You think: "Forget it. It's not worth it."

You were going great, and then everything just fell apart. So what happened? Why did the scale stop moving down?

There are many reasons why weight loss plateaus, but one mistake I see repeatedly is people don't stop to ask themselves what the end really looks like. If you don't know exactly where you want to go, how will you know when you're there?

People tell me, "Michelle, I will just know when I'm there." That's not true. I can't tell you how many people have lost the weight they said they wanted to lose, then looked in the mirror at the size they wrote on paper was their goal, and still not loved what they saw and how they felt.

Your mind needs a clear picture of where it is headed so it can begin releasing the layers of protection it has built up over the years. And, when you have a clear vision of where you want to go, you will know when you're there. You will be able to feel and see it.

To get there, though, you have to sit down and ask yourself what you want. Not just what size do you want to be, but how do you want to feel? What sort of life do you want to live?

When you picture your ideal body you also must picture your ideal life, because to attain the body, you must begin living that life. Once you do, the weight just falls off. More importantly, you get the results you want – the real results, not just the smaller body – way before the scale gets to where you think you want it to go.

Can you imagine letting go of your obsession to have a certain body? Allowing yourself to visualize the life you want to live and then starting to live it immediately? So that the size of your body is just an added bonus?

Most of my clients don't have that big, "I did it!" reaction because they started feeling amazing long before the weight came off. By the time they reach their weight loss goals, it's just icing on the metaphorical cake.

This is the most pleasant way to release weight. It's also the quickest. But, it takes the largest amount of commitment because you have to be willing to make massive life changes, no matter how scary they are.

Homework Assignment #4
Picturing Your Ideal Life

Sit down, with your feet pressed firmly to the floor. Begin focusing on your breath, paying attention to each inhale and exhale. Follow the breath with your thoughts for a few moments, until your mind is blank and ready to work. Then, picture your ideal body and life. Bring in all the senses to make this visualization real.

Where are you? What are you doing? Who are you with? What feelings do you get from the environment around you? What does that environment look like? What smells, tastes, sounds do you experience?

Allow your entire body to fill with the emotion of having everything you desire and more. Connect to this vision as much as you need to, and allow it to override any fears of becoming it. Keep it in mind in the days ahead.

Setting the Stage

Visualization can be tough, especially for beginners. Listening to guided meditation tapes or simply sitting quietly and focusing on your breath for a few minutes several days in a row can help get you in the right mindset to attempt this exercise. Make sure you're in an environment where you feel relaxed and supported. Consider dimming the lights or turning on some ocean waves or light music to calm your nerves. Make sure you're physically comfortable, and then allow yourself to start dreaming.

Working Harder Only Amplifies Your Current Results, It Does Not Change Them

As discussed previously, there often comes a point in our weight loss journeys when the scale stops moving, our weight plateaus, and we stop seeing progress. Sometimes this is because we haven't fully visualized where we want to go. Sometimes, we just get tired.

We decide we want to sleep in, or that we really want to eat out, or we attend a social event and overindulge with delicious food. At that point, it's as if everything we started goes down the toilet, and we feel we have to work even harder to make up for it. We decide to go to the gym twice as often, and to focus on our calories even more.

But, the crazy thing is, when we put in all that effort and work really hard at losing weight, we will always get to a point where the results stop, even without temptations.

The reason why it stops working, the reason it's so hard to resist temptation and why you hit up against resistance every time, is because the method in which you chose to lose weight sucks. Instead of working harder, you need to let go.

TIP: Doing more of the same thing harder does not get you the results you want.

Doing more of the same thing, only gets you more of what you've already gotten.

Upset because you went on a food bender after cutting your caloric intake to 1500 for 30 days? Cutting it to 1200 isn't going to help you lose weight. It's only going to make you binge eat again, sooner this time.

Frustrated because you worked out four days a week for six weeks and saw the scale drop and drop, but now it's stuck? Upping your time at the gym isn't going to fix the problem long term. You may see the scale drop a little at first, but you'll likely plateau again, and even faster.

If your current program or diet isn't working, it doesn't matter how much harder you work at it, it won't work long term. And, for those of you who think temporary results mean it's working, you are mistaken.

TIP: Temporary results will always be temporary. Therefore, whatever you do to get them doesn't work.

Get honest with yourself. What does work for your body? Think back to times in your life when your body effortlessly improved, when you "just got smaller" or maintained your optimum weight without trying. Those are the instances in which however you were being worked.

If you don't have those examples in your life, look at other people. People who live effortlessly in their ideal bodies do not force themselves to go to the gym; eat low-calorie, frozen foods; and forgo social events so they don't eat up all the delicious appetizers. They don't cut out food and work doubly hard when they are tired.

These are your models, *not* people who are dieting for life. Not people who have lost a tremendous amount of weight in a manner one never would want to maintain.

If your results are not consistent, doing whatever you are doing more or harder will just get you more inconsistent results.

It's important to note here that obtaining a small size doesn't necessarily mean your program or diet is working, just as not obtaining that size doesn't mean it's not. It isn't about the size, or the number on the scale. It's about how you feel. Getting down to the small size or the low weight doesn't mean anything if you still look at yourself and only see fat.

Do you feel like what you are doing is working? Do you feel happy and confident in your body? Does it do what you want it to do?

Your emotions play a big role in determining whether something is working. I have had clients come to me who hadn't yet lost the weight they said they wanted to lose, but they confessed to feeling so much lighter and freer.

If you feel this way, does it really matter what the scale says?

I'm not saying you should settle for a physical body that doesn't serve you, just that you should consider how you are measuring your results. Are you basing your feelings and thoughts about your body on a label and a hunk of metal or on the way you feel in your own skin?

In a private coaching session, one of my clients told me how desperately she just wanted to be able to go to the store, grab clothes off the rack, and have them look amazing. I told her to go do it now! The very next day she came back beaming, happy to report that she was able to do just that.

Now, obviously she didn't lose weight in 24 hours so why the sudden shift in her experience?

She began to see and think about herself differently. Instead of focusing on the size of her clothes, she focused on how she felt. And, because she started to feel lighter from the minute we began our work together, she was able to view her physical appearance as lighter, too.

TIP: When you change what you think, you change what you see.

Are you so attached to a number on a scale or on a tag that you can't allow yourself to feel instant gratification?

Most people come to me because they want to feel different. They assume that to feel different they must look different. This couldn't be further from the truth.

It's not to say you can't desire an alternate physical body than your current one, as everyone is entitled to whatever they want without explanation. However, there is absolutely no reason to delay the feelings you wish to feel and tie them to a physical body.

Your body doesn't have to dictate your emotions. You can and should feel fabulous right now. In fact, allowing yourself to feel great now will speed up your weight loss process by quickly moving you into your ideal life. And, once you're living your ideal life, getting your ideal body becomes as easy as breathing.

Homework Assignment #5
Visualize Your Ideal Body

Take an inventory of your weight experience and write down all the different bodies you have experienced. Try to go as far back as you can. When was the first time you remember thinking you needed to lose weight?

Then, look for the times when you got results. For the purposes of this exercise, you can include both temporary results and the times when your body was smaller and you don't believe you did anything to influence it being smaller. Start to look for clues about what was going on in your life when you were in the most ideal body to you.

If you don't have any of these experiences, find someone who you view is living in their ideal body, and ask them what they believe they are doing to maintain their results.

For Example:

You may have been very busy in college, too busy to worry about your weight. You were working, going to school, and trying to figure out your life. Yet, when you think back on it, you realize you started to drop weight at this time in your life, without any type of diet. Consider how you may be able to re-create the feelings you had then about not focusing on your weight, since you know that has worked for you in the past.

Setting the Stage

Even if you don't have a time in your life when you effortlessly lost weight, you can still get a lot out of this assignment. There are most likely situations that you can remember when you didn't struggle. Step back into those moments and dig deep to discover who you were as a person at that time.

What positive attributes did you have then? What similarities and differences can you find between then and now? (Besides your age, silly.)

We can learn so much from ourselves. Take the time to be your own teacher.

Results Affirmations
(Pin these to your mirror, car, or anywhere they'll be seen regularly.)

I am a success, regardless of my weight loss results.

The easiest way to shift into getting the results I desire is to be here, now.

As I move through my journey to having what I desire, I will stay in this moment and simply breathe.

When I let go of all that I am not, I will finally step into all that I am meant to become.

I am always on a journey and will not get distracted by the end results.

Being One with Your Body

Getting your ideal body isn't about what you do, it's about how you think, feel, and act. It's about who you are. To get the body you truly want, you must become one with the body you have now.

Your Excess Weight is Here for a Reason, and It's Never About the Weight

When I gained 25 pounds and tons of body fat in my early twenties, while working out two times a day, seven days a week; restricting myself to a 1200-calorie diet; and substituting with artificial sweeteners, I was completely bewildered.

I went from being a "naturally" thin person who never really thought about my weight to someone completely obsessed. I couldn't figure out what had gone wrong, and I was upset.

And, as the pounds kept creeping on, I couldn't help but ask myself, "Why is this happening to me?"

You've probably asked yourself the same thing. You've probably also been really angry about your weight gain. Angry that you don't have what you want, and that you can't figure out why.

Let me tell you a secret: There is a why. The truth is you gained weight for a reason, and it's nothing your body did to you. You aren't being punished, and you're not a victim. In fact, it's just the opposite. Your body is motivating you to change into who you are meant to become.

TIP: Your weight isn't happening to you, it's happening for you.

My weight gain gave me my purpose for being on the planet. Without that experience, I never would have begun teaching about weight loss in the way I have. I never would have been so blessed to see how much change I help people bring about in their own lives. Those 25 pounds were the best thing that ever happened to me.

You may wonder why you have to gain weight to experience such a transformation. "Isn't there an easier way to change?" you might ask. Maybe, but think about it: How many crazy-town schemes have you tried to lose weight? Consider how many beliefs, values, morals, habits, and stuck points you have burst through in your effort to get results.

One of the most beautiful things about weight gain is its extreme power of motivation.

When you can see something physically on your body, you are very motivated to change. Nothing else has quite the same effect. Unfortunately, many of us take the wrong actions, and make the wrong changes, to lose the weight.

We think it's about how much we eat, how often we exercise, or what kind of activities we do. It's not. The changes we have to make are major life changes that lead to huge transformations: leaving an unfulfilling relationship, starting a business, standing in our own power, cutting off ties with toxic people, and letting go of false but deeply held beliefs. The trick is to use the motivation to lose weight to make these changes, and finally live the lives we truly desire.

Your weight is here to teach you something. You must learn and live the lesson. You must fully change and step into your life in every way that you currently aren't. If you have ever done any type of transformation work you will know that the biggest transformations take place when you let go of all the stuff in your life that isn't serving you.

When I wasn't getting the results I desired in my life I knew I had to hire help. When I began working with my coach and healer it became very clear I was going to have to let go of a relationship that wasn't serving me. It was causing me a tremendous amount of stress and frustration. It was draining and holding me back from bringing my truth to the world.

I was afraid to let it go because I didn't want to let the other person down and because letting it go meant letting go of my income associated with it, which meant that I would immediately have to replace that revenue stream.

I tried to half-ass let it go. I sort of exited the relationship, but I didn't really let it go. The universe gave me more symptoms and reasons to truly let it go. Finally I completely released the relationship, both personally and professionally.

Once I did, I began sleeping at night. I let go of frustration and stress. I felt at peace even with all the fears around finances. I also began receiving opportunities left and right to help me along my path.

I would notice this a lot with my friends and romantic relationships, too. They would be in toxic relationships with men who didn't treat them right, and they knew they had to get out. When we would talk about it, they would say: "I'm waiting for the right guy to show up but there is no point of letting this one go in the meantime. If a great opportunity comes, I will dump this guy and move on."

Isn't it funny how this rarely happens? None of my friends had Prince Charming show up while still in the toxic relationship. They would finally get fed up, leave the guys, and that's when their future spouses would show up.

I can promise you, you will never have easy, automatic weight maintenance until you change your life in every area that you are currently settling. Just as Mr. or Ms. Right won't show up as long as you're holding on to Mr. or Ms.

Wrong, your body is not going to change until you stop settling for less than you deserve. But you don't have to struggle when making these changes. The universe will completely support you in your transitions, if you let it.

TIP: The universe rewards and supports you through tough decisions.

I have seen it happen for myself and my clients often. When you are in alignment and willing to let go of everything in your life that isn't serving you, you will be supported and will receive exceptional results.

The only reason you wouldn't is if you allow yourself to get in your own way (been there, too)! If you psych yourself out and believe in lack over abundance, then you will struggle. Stay in a place of peace, and you will be in the flow of life and will receive every day.

Homework Assignment #6
My Weight Gain Lessons

You must understand why your weight is here. What lessons are you meant to learn and where do you need to step up in your life? Where are you settling or surviving? What action steps do you need to take immediately to have the most incredible, fulfilling life?

Write it all out and begin finding gratitude for your weight for teaching you these life lessons. Practice gratitude every morning and night.

For Example:

Perhaps you are aware that you are "getting through" your days. Why aren't you experiencing more joy? What are you tolerating in your life that you could be letting go? Where are you settling? How can you begin to share the gift of fully living with your body more?

Setting the Stage

Be open and honest about what gifts your weight could possibly give you.

What major life lessons have you learned so far? What have you learned not to do? What fears do you have about being open and honest?

Acknowledge that you may feel shame or embarrassment and that's okay. Start with where you are.

Your Desire to Lose Weight Isn't About Your Weight

Most of you may think that your issue with your weight revolves around the fact that you have excess weight. In other words, you may believe that this "issue with excess weight" will be solved simply by removing the excess weight.

Problem solved, right? Wrong.

The truth is your weight is closely tied to your body image, your relationship with your body.

Think about it:

Why do you have such a STRONG desire to lose weight? What if you had excess weight and didn't NEED to lose it? Or, what if you were the only person on the planet? If there were no other people to judge you or compare yourself to, would you still have such a strong desire to lose weight? Or would you shift your focus elsewhere?

Unfortunately, we live in a society in which loving and accepting your body can be perceived as weird, and in which we have been told that perfect is better than real. Someone who is holding onto a little excess weight and loves herself anyway can be looked down upon. People may assume she is lazy, eats fast food all day, or is not taking care of herself. And, when given a photo of her to compare to a size two, photo-shopped model, many will say the model is more attractive and beautiful – even though the tiny woman in that second picture doesn't actually exist in the real world. But, it is the first woman whom we should model ourselves after.

Most of us are unhappy with our bodies, and it is because of our focus on an ideal that doesn't even exist. We pinch and prod our bodies, cringing at every ounce of fat. We tell ourselves that if we removed the excess fat and there was nothing left to pinch, then we would be perfect and beautiful.

But, even if we did manage to remove the fat, and became model thin, we still wouldn't be good enough. We still wouldn't look like the model in the picture, because *she* doesn't even look like that. Computer imaging and retouching have completely stolen our vision of what real, healthy people look like. Yet, even once we know that, even when we are intellectually aware that our ideals are unrealistic, it is tremendously difficult to move past them.

In our society we have been conditioned to always seek more growth. This drive for improvement doesn't allow us to sit comfortably in front of somebody else and say, "I love myself just as I am." Instead, we feel judged, knowing that maybe in their minds everyone in the world should be a size 2. And, then we feel uncomfortable saying we are okay with our softer, curvier frames.

We also have people around us who share their judgments of our bodies out loud, either behind our backs or to our faces. These comments can push us toward believing we need to change our bodies to fit other people's ideals, and our goal becomes making those around us comfortable instead of admitting what would make us comfortable.

Can you be a model with your softer, curvier frame? Maybe, maybe not, but likely you have created a life for yourself where you don't need to be a model. Is there anything wrong with not wanting to be a model? Or not desiring a model's body? *What if you designed a life where you are so loving and kind to yourself that you don't need a perfect body to compensate for anything?* Would you still feel you needed to lose weight?

I have heard all sorts of responses to this argument. People tell me: "But Michelle, what about people who are extremely overweight? It's so bad for their health! You can't possibly tell them to accept their bodies as they are." To which I reply, "I absolutely can."

There is no rule anywhere that states that if you are overweight you must in turn hate your body. In fact, if someone with excess weight decided to show her body love, her body would have no choice but to release weight because **part of self-love is self-care, and the body doesn't become overweight without some type of lack of love and care.** In other words, nobody I know has ever "loved their body fat."

Nobody I know has ever decided to completely call off the war inside of him, let go of all his hatred and judgments, fallen completely in love with his self, and then gained a bunch of weight. So tell me, what is the harm?

Homework Assignment #7
Connecting to My True Body Desires

What would your ideal body be if there were no other people on the planet to judge you? What body would allow you to live out your purpose and mission and allow you to live free from control of your body, weight, and food/exercise? How would it feel? What could it do?

Setting the Stage

We tend to crave rock-hard abs and toned arms so that others can see our accomplishments. The drive for hard, muscular bodies with low body fat isn't about how those bodies serve us. It's about competition. Think of what life would be like if there were no other people to compare your body to. No celebrities prancing around at 50 years old, looking hotter than a teenager. Imagine it's just you, and your own personal preferences.

Perfection Will Never Guarantee Happiness

I ask you the following question and I want you to think very seriously about it: What are you afraid will happen if you love and accept your body as it is?

Push through the old belief system that may be telling you that if you do accept and love yourself you won't eat healthy and move, because it's not true. Loving and accepting yourself doesn't equal channel surfing and eating bon-bons 10 hours a day. In fact, I bet you'd be hard pressed to find a time in your life when you ever gained weight because you decided to love and accept yourself.

Self-love and self-care lead to weight loss, not weight gain. If you can't learn how to love and accept your body just as it is, then you will continue to chase an impossible dream. Impossible because even if you reach the goal you set for yourself, you still won't have learned to love yourself. And even though you believe a thinner you equals a more lovable you, I am here to tell you it's just not true.

Perfection will never create peace. You think if you have the perfect body you will in turn have the perfect life. I assure you it's not true.

In fact, perfection creates the opposite of peace. It creates restriction, deprivation, rules, and frustration. It fixes an impossible ideal in your mind, which you chase each and every day, all while telling yourself that where you are is not okay. You imagine that once you achieve this "perfect" body, you will stop being criticized. You believe perfection means you will never be judged.

That, my friends, is a big, fat lie.

You will always be judged. You will always be criticized by the people around you who are quite simply not okay where they are. And, if you are using weight loss as a vehicle to escape judgment, you are slowly crawling up a never-ending hill.

Instead of taking it personally when someone comments on your weight, understand their comments are not about you. They stem from the commenter's own personal insecurities and hang-ups. Do not allow them to make you judge yourself. Instead, continue to practice self-love and self-care by finding out what nourishes you.

Nourishing the Body is Loving the Self

From the time we are infants, nourishment equals love. We are nourished by our mothers' milk, our fathers' laughter, our grandparents' hugs, our cozy beds. As we get older, it becomes our jobs to nourish ourselves in the same ways we were nourished as children, with food, fun, love, and rest. We cannot feel nourished, however, if we aren't open to receiving nourishment.

You may have noticed self-sabotaging behavior with food, exercise, rest, and play. You may find that you talk yourself out of the very things you know will allow you to feel nourished or that you force yourself to do things that aren't nourishing.

If you don't love your body and want to take care of it, you're not going to participate in nourishing activities. You will talk yourself into overeating and talk yourself out of fun movement. You will tell yourself you don't have enough time to rest or stop yourself from resting even when you are finally slowing down.

You also will lie to yourself about play, telling yourself either that you don't have enough time, you don't have hobbies, or that all you want to do is drink wine and watch TV. Now trust me, I love me some wine and TV, but only when I choose to participate in both of those activities, not when I fall into them because there is nothing else to do. Or not because I am on auto-pilot and two hours and a bottle of wine just magically disappeared.

Bringing presence to your relationship with your body will allow you to get honest about nourishment. Do you love yourself enough to receive nourishment? Are you allowing yourself to feel nourished through various activities? Once you know the answers to these questions, your relationship with your body and your body image will dramatically improve.

Homework Assignment #8
Finding Out What Nourishes You

Take a moment to consider what nourishes you. Ask yourself what makes you feel really good. What activities do you find most rewarding? What foods and places make you feel warm, safe, and protected? What gives you energy? What makes you feel enthused and full of joy? Write it down somewhere you can refer back to when you catch yourself engaging in an activity that doesn't nourish who you are.

Setting the Stage

Don't get caught up in the how right now. Just bring presence to your life and your body. Don't worry about implementation. When you hear the self-sabotaging thoughts, stop and breathe. Ask yourself what you really need in that moment.

Master Communication with Your Body for Maximum Results

Are you in tune with your intuition? You know that little voice that tells you what to do and what not to do? Where do you think it comes from?

Where do you think an artist gets his ideas to paint? How about a musician? Where does she get the idea of how to put a song together? A writer? Where does she come up with her next science fiction novel? Intuition.

They each feel their intuition guiding them, and they each express it in their own way.

TIP: You have this guidance and intuition within your body. It already knows how to be ideal. It's already inside of you.

It's talking to you every day, telling you what to do and what not to do. You are either not hearing it or you are ignoring it.

When you eat something and get sick, your body is telling you to stop eating that.

When you feel high after a run, your body is telling you it loves that.

When you get a random idea to join Zumba, your body is telling you it wants it.

When you decide that pizza sounds like the most delicious thing for dinner, your body wants it.

The beautiful thing is even if you get it wrong, and instead of your intuition it was your old patterns trying to sabotage your success, you will get a strong negative reaction to it, and you will know for next time.

So let's say you get an idea to order pizza. You aren't sure if your body is just craving pizza or your mind is trying to trick you into staying the same. So you order the pizza and eat it. Turns out it's not all that satisfying and/or you get sick after you eat it. You know your body would never voluntarily get sick, so you know the idea didn't come from your intuition. As long as you recognize this and adjust, your intuition will get louder and louder and you will barely hear those self-sabotaging thoughts.

This same thing applies to thoughts and ideas from outside sources. You always want to test any advice and information with your intuition. Does it feel right to you? Does it feel like beliefs or principles you want to live by for life? If so, great! Run with it. If not, throw it away!

Homework Assignment #9
Intuitive Living

Practice one full day of doing everything that "little voice" tells you to do, without any judgment.

If it wants you to say something, just say it. If it wants you to eat something, eat it. Move in a certain way or skip your workout? Do it.

See how it feels to only go by intuition without considering what the "experts" say. See what feels good and what doesn't feel good. If you decide to skip the gym, does it feel amazing to rest or crappy because deep down you wanted to move?

Don't get down on yourself if you make a "wrong" decision. The purpose of this exercise is to reopen communication between you and your body, not to open the door to guilt or blame. Enjoy and have fun!

Setting the Stage

Most of us fear living from our intuitive voice, and it's almost always due to what others may think or feel. For example, you may hear your intuition tell you to set a boundary with someone at work, but you are worried if you say something they may not like you. Or maybe your voice really wants to eat pasta instead of salad, but you are worried that if someone sees you eat pasta they may think you don't want to lose weight and aren't trying hard enough. I challenge you to completely let go of what the world thinks of you. Live by your own rules. People will always judge others but it's never really about you, it's about them. Listen to your body.

Body Affirmations
(Pin these to your mirror, car, or anywhere they'll be seen regularly.)

I listen to my body.

My body has strength, endurance, and health.

My body is perfect, right now, as it is.

Confidence, radiance, and happiness are my choice.

My body is not punishing me with weight; it's communicating with me.

Being One with Food

It's easy to blame food for your current weight, but food is not the cause of your weight gain. Lots of people eat low quality food or foods high in calories and fats every day and are thin. Others eat nothing but low-calorie entrees and snacks and are still overweight. Some were once able to eat whatever they wanted without worrying about their weight, and now can't. Others continue to eat according to their cravings and needs their entire lives. Why?

Food doesn't choose favorites; it doesn't choose certain people for whom calories mean more and other people for whom they mean less. The difference isn't in who you are or what you eat. **It's in what you think about what you eat.**

Everything we put in our bodies has to be digested and metabolized for energy. Generally, this is a normal process that works exactly as it should. But, when we're afraid, anxious, or stressed, it changes things. It creates a toxic environment that then renders only toxic results.

If you want to lose weight, it is absolutely crucial that your meal times are stress free, relaxed, and fun.

If you want your ideal body, you must have ideal digestion and metabolism. Instead of cutting out food, cut out stress while you eat. Create enjoyable meal times by slowing down and staying present during your meals. Sit down to eat, and savor every bite. Express gratitude for the abundance on your plate and in your life.

Your external world is a reflection of your internal world. So take food off the chopping block and turn inward:

What is going on when you eat?

What are your beliefs around food before, during, and after your meal?

What kinds of foods are you drawn to eat? Why?

How do you feel before, during, and after a meal? When you eat certain foods? When you follow your cravings?

If you are drawn to low quality food every day, focus on changing who you are being. It's you, not the food. Valuing yourself more will automatically trigger you to want to fill your body with higher quality, nourishing food.

TIP: When you change on the inside, you will automatically change on the outside.

Homework Assignment #10
Food Inventory Log

Get out a piece of paper and make a food inventory log. Use it for no more than seven days. (If it begins to feel restrictive, do not do it more than one day!) Include the following:

Type of meal. It's not important what you eat, so don't measure, manage, or control. Just write down if it is breakfast, lunch, dinner, or a snack. No judgment on what you are eating.

How long it took you to eat it. It's important to notice how fast you are eating. Ideal metabolism requires slow eating with plenty of time for digestion.

How full you are. After you eat, measure how full you are on a 1 to 10 scale. Seven would be optimal, and 10 would be stuffed.

How much pleasure you received from eating. Again, use a 1 – 10 scale. 10 would be ideal.

How much satisfaction you received from eating. Again, 10 would be ideal. Notice whether you liked what you ate, and if it felt satisfying to you.

Your goal with this is to slow down, savor, and appreciate the opportunity to nourish yourself.

For Example:

Breakfast - 10 min. - 6 - 7 - 7
Lunch - 15 min. - 7 - 8 - 9
Dinner - 20 min. - 7 - 10 - 9

Setting the Stage

When doing this exercise, you must stay present. You won't know how to answer the questions if you are worrying about bills or your grocery list.

Remove distractions, stay focused, and concentrate on eating. Only then will you have the most accurate representation of what is going on for you.

Food is Just Food, Until You Determine Its Caloric Value

We are very calorie focused in our country. Instead of considering what we want to eat or what our body needs when we want to lose weight, we focus on what has the fewest calories. This is absurd.

By this logic, eating a doughnut for breakfast is better than eating a bagel, because the doughnut has fewer calories. No matter that the bagel will keep you full longer, or that the doughnut will deliver a mighty sugar crash within hours of eating it. As this example shows, food choices are about a lot more than calories. So, what's with our obsession with these pesky little numbers?

The truth is they sound pleasant. They give us an easy-to-follow weight loss formula, all wrapped up with a neat little bow. We count how many calories we eat, and as long as we don't eat more than we burn, we never gain weight. We appreciate the simplicity, and we love the illusion of control the formula gives us – but that's all it is, an illusion, because, as we discussed earlier, the formula doesn't work.

You still may be feeling some resistance to this idea. That's okay. It's hard to give up the illusion of control. At some point, though, you will have to realize that control is almost always an illusion. In life, there just isn't much that we can control, including our weight. This also is okay, **because releasing control will give you far greater results than the caloric formula ever could**.

Instead of clinging to a formula that doesn't work, try reimagining how you view food. I like to teach my clients that all food is 0 calories until you begin adding calories, which – in our calorie-obsessed culture – most of us do all the time.

When you say, "This pizza is so bad for me, it's going to go right to my hips," you have just made that slice of pizza worth 500 calories. When you change your thoughts and say, "Wow, this pizza is so delicious, this is amazing!" instead, you have just subtracted 500 calories.

Once you change your thought patterns, you stop determining the caloric value of food with negative thoughts and judgments. Then, food will just be food and you will allow yourself to enjoy it. For some of you, that will be enough to release all your weight. For others, there will be healing to be done in other areas too, but at least you get to enjoy food again.

Homework Assignment #11
Change Your Relationship with Food

Catch yourself when you begin assigning caloric values to food. Notice when you begin speaking about food as the contributor to your weight. Then, ask yourself, "Is this the relationship I want to have with food for the rest of my life?" When the answer is "No," don't pass judgment on yourself. Just gently correct the thought pattern. Remind yourself that food is just food. Then, follow your intuition and eat what feels right to you at that moment. Make sure to acknowledge the pleasure you get from eating!

For example:

You're at a dinner party, and a bowl of rolls is being passed around. You can smell the delicious sourdough aroma and can imagine how delicious it would taste. You're feeling highly motivated to take one of these rolls and enjoy every bite, but then you remind yourself that you don't need the extra carbs, that you are trying to lower your carbs to lose weight, and so you start to pass the bowl without taking one.

Then, you stop. You realize you've just assigned calories to the rolls that they don't have. You gently remind yourself that food is just food, and that you can and should eat what your body is saying it wants. So, you grab one, and eat it with full pleasure, enjoyment, and satisfaction, knowing you are honoring your body by enjoying the food it needs.

Setting the Stage

If you've been hopping from one weight loss program to another, denying yourself what you want may feel more natural than indulging in your body's desires. But, remember, to lose weight for good you must act and think like you are already in your ideal body. If you had never had a weight problem would you take the roll?

Most people would say yes. I bet you are one of them. And, I'd guess that if you were operating from an ideal weight consciousness, instead of an overweight consciousness, you'd have taken the roll, no stress or guilt about it.

If you want to be someone who can easily eat a roll with no stress in the world, it's time to start practicing. Agree to take the roll the next time you want it. No more punishing. To get the life and body you want, you must begin making decisions as if you already have them. (For more information on this, see the next section.)

You Must Eat Like You Are Already In Your Ideal Body

One of the biggest mistakes I see traditional weight loss programs make is teaching people to alter their food to lose weight. This will only work if the alterations you are making feel good and effortless and like something you desire to maintain for the rest of your life. If this is not the case, stop what you are doing immediately!

TIP: You must eat the way you intend to eat forever.

When I ask my clients, "How would you eat if you were at your goal weight?" most tell me they would automatically eat fruits and veggies, and that they wouldn't judge or deny themselves if they wanted a slice of pizza. They describe a beautiful relationship with food. One in which they honor their body by fueling it with healthy and nutritious foods, and by following their intuition.

This may worry you. You may think you couldn't do this, that you can't eat as if you were in your ideal body, because you would "lack willpower" and eat nothing but "junk." You may worry that without consciously controlling every bite that passes your lips, you will only pack on more pounds.

This is a false belief. I've never had a client tell me that at his or her goal weight he or she would eat fast food every day. And, I've never seen that happen either.

When you are envisioning your ideal body, you are seeing a healthier, better version of your current body. This includes the quality of the food you are feeding it.

If you have been depriving yourself of certain foods over the years, your vision might look different, but don't panic. Your initial vision is not your forever eating style; you just need to get back in balance.

When I first went off of dieting I wanted to eat out every meal, because I had forbid it for so long. I indulged myself in this, and it wasn't long before my priorities shifted. As soon as I wasn't denying myself what I wanted, I started wanting different things. Within a short period of time, I couldn't even fathom eating out as much anymore. I just wanted delicious home-cooked food that was high quality and pleasurable.

To eat like you would in your ideal body, you must remove all judgment and act out of intuition. This takes trust.

You must listen to your body no matter what it says. If it says it wants pizza, eat it and then see how much pleasure and satisfaction you get. If it's a lot, you know that pizza is something your body enjoys and should have. If you find that it's a little disappointing and that it gives you a stomachache, then it is probably a good idea to lessen the amount of pizza you eat to serve your body in the highest way.

If you find yourself in the latter category, though, know that this doesn't mean you can't eat pizza. It only means that you are going to have negative consequences if you do.

Sometimes it's worth it anyway. Most of the time it's not, but this is for your body to decide. Listen to it and follow its advice. It knows what it needs.

Homework Assignment #12
Connecting to Your True Eating Desires

Get to a quiet place and focus on your breath. Envision your ideal body and ask yourself how you would eat if you were already in it.

In this vision, how do you feel about food? How do you act around food? What do you want? What do you eat?

Then, ask yourself what are the major differences you see in your vision versus your current reality? Make a committed decision to eat like you are in your ideal body every day.

Setting the Stage

In order to get real, truthful answers in this exercise, you must eliminate any guilt or shame.

Be honest with yourself about how you see your life with food in your ideal body. What is included? What is not included? If a particular food triggers feelings of guilt or shame, ask yourself why. What beliefs underlie those feelings? Whose voice are you hearing when you tell yourself not to eat something or that it is "bad" for you? If it isn't yours, try to release the voice and the negative patterns, and replace them with more positive ones, such as "I am honoring my body by giving it what it needs" or "I trust myself."

Once you are clear about how you would eat in your ideal body, you are now capable of changing your lifelong patterns. Be aware, though, that old eating habits and thought patterns may creep up. When they do, release them without judgment. It's up to you to stay focused on what you really want.

Food Feeds Your Mind and Your Stomach

If you are struggling with overeating, then this will be the most profound section to you. I struggled with overeating and had absolutely no idea how to stop it, until I learned this information.

We are aware that we feed our stomachs. We can feel the food in our bellies, and we understand how it moves through the body. For these reasons, most weight loss methods dealing with overeating focus on the stomach. These programs focus on portion control, eating until some percentage of "fullness" is achieved, and curtailing or shrinking appetite. These methods won't work to end overeating for good, though, because overeating isn't a problem with your stomach. It's a problem with your mind.

Eating is not just a way to create energy. Along with feeding our stomachs, we feed our brains. We receive **P**leasure, **S**atisfaction, **F**ulfillment, **N**ourishment, **C**omfort, and many other emotions from eating. These experiences, which are felt and realized in the mind, are a crucial part of eating in general.

If we are not getting the emotional experiences we need when eating, we will continue to eat until we get them or until we become so full we are sick. This is the basis of overeating and binge eating.

TIP: When we don't get our emotional vitamins, our mind will guide us to get more food until we do.

Instead of feeling guilty or judging yourself when you've been binging, ask yourself how you can feel satisfaction, fulfillment, nourishment, or comfort in that moment. What do you need to do once you have already eaten and you realize you missed out on all those emotions?

What gives you pleasure? Maybe it's a hot bath or a conversation with a friend. Maybe it's a book or a cup of hot tea. Maybe you need to take a walk or go dancing. Maybe you need to start or finish a project you've been delaying. You even may need something else to eat; the answer depends on you.

Once again, take a moment to tune in to your intuition. Listen to your body. Then, give it what it needs. Do this each time you realize you've eaten without getting your emotional vitamins. Slowing down to eat and creating a relaxing eating environment will help you both derive positive experiences from your food and notice more promptly when you haven't gotten them.

Homework Assignment #13
The Slow Eating Challenge

Homework assignment number 10 taught you how to pay attention to how much pleasure, satisfaction, nourishment, comfort, and fulfillment you get out of each meal. Now, it is time to think about how to maximize those emotions and experiences.

At your next meal, challenge yourself to eat as slowly as possible. Notice every flavor, herb, and spice. Put down the fork after each bite, and savor the textures and flavors in your mouth. Take deep breaths and let the food fill you up.

As you eat, check in with yourself frequently. How are you feeling? Do you like the food you are eating? Are you getting your emotional vitamins P, S, F, N, and C? If not, what can you do to enhance the experience?

Eventually, this all will become an unconscious experience. In the beginning, however, it takes conscious effort to create a different mealtime. It gets easier with practice, so feel free to undertake this assignment as many times as necessary until you notice a change.

Setting the Stage

For this assignment, you should set up the most relaxing eating environment you can think of. Do you like candles? Dim the lights and set some out. Lay out a nice tablecloth. Turn on your favorite light music. Feel free to use the fancy dishes and nice napkins. Pour a glass of wine, if that helps you savor each moment.

Eliminate any distractions and experiment with closing your eyes and turning up your other senses. Let this exercise be the door to a new relationship with food forever.

Food Affirmations
(Pin these to your mirror, car, or anywhere they'll be seen regularly.)

Food is just food, not the vehicle that causes my body to gain weight.

Food eaten with full pleasure, relaxation, and satisfaction is calorie free.

My food quality is my declaration of how much I love and value myself.

All food is equal until I decide it doesn't work for my body.

Food causes positive emotional experiences and can be celebrated with joy.

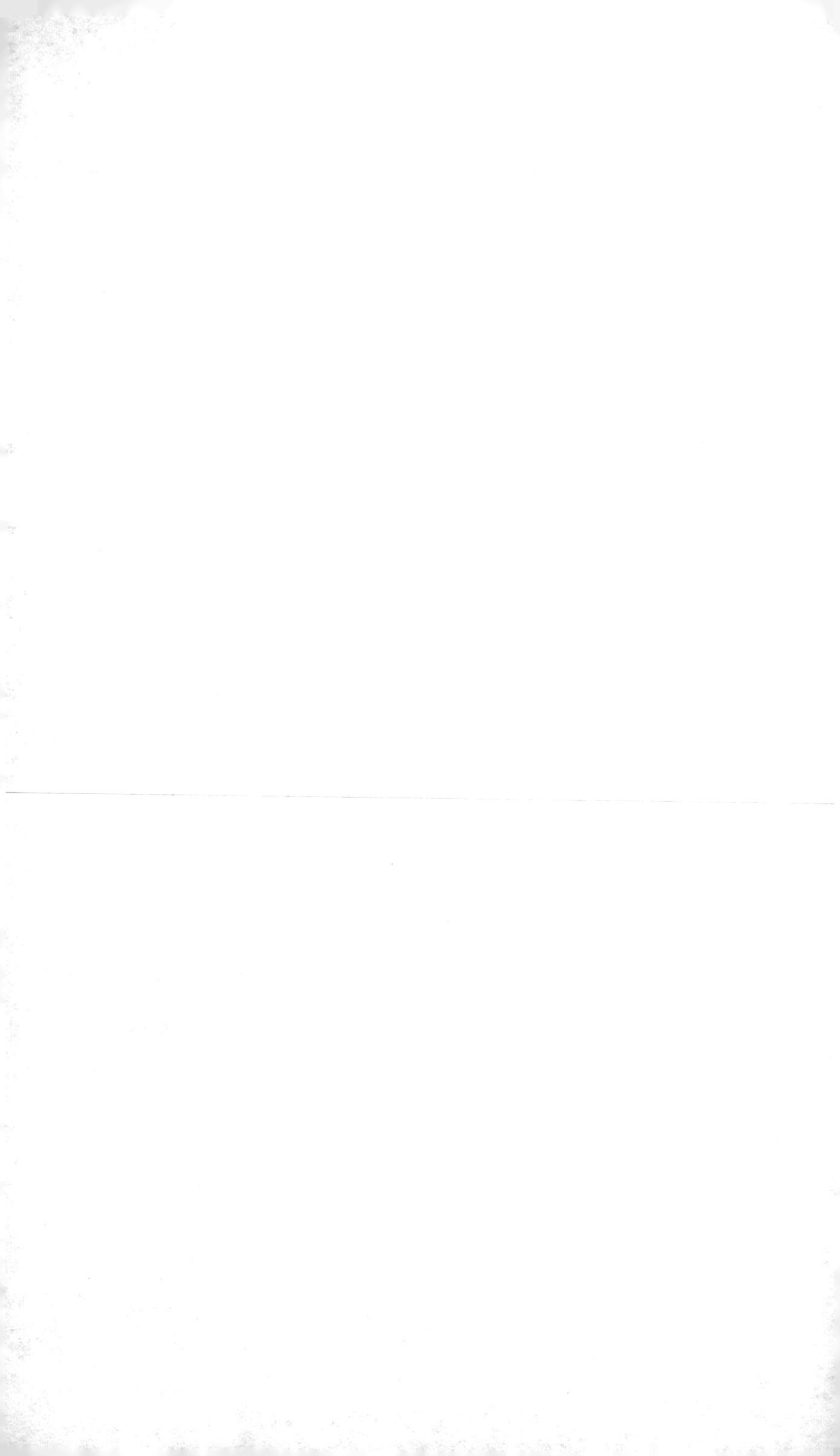

Being One with Movement

Many people who struggle with their weight view movement as a punishment. They see it as something they "have to do" to "make up for" eating the things they feel badly about or for not fitting into the size they think they should fit into. This is at odds with our natural state as human beings.

Movement is what helps us experience life. It enables us to try new things, to reach new heights. It is a way to challenge our bodies and to grow from that challenge. It offers us confidence and affirms our self-worth. No wonder viewing it negatively makes us view ourselves in a harsh light!

Movement is an indication that we are alive and energetic. It's a representation of our health and abilities. If you can run three miles or hold a warrior pose for 3 to 5 minutes, then you know you can deal with a bad breakup or losing your job.

A healthy, strong, vibrant body that moves with ease and flow is one of the most beautiful gifts we can give ourselves. Allow it to be just that.

TIP: You don’t have to be an athlete.

Movement should be fun; something you do for you because you want to do it. If what you really want is to run a marathon, great! Go out and train for it. But, if (like me) you think that sounds agonizing, don’t do it. Who cares if you can run 28 miles or not? Who cares if you can hike to the top of a mountain? Not everyone is meant to accomplish these tasks, and that’s perfectly fine.

Allow yourself to just be yourself. Let go of an idealized version of a superhero where you can do everything. Focus on your specific gifts and desires only. What do you want to do?

Homework Assignment #14
My Intuitive Movement

Sit down with pen and paper and dream about what your life is meant to be. What did you want to do when you were a kid? What would you do if you had endless amounts of money or health? Without limitations, what are your true desires?

Now check that list to see what types of activities are on it. Is climbing a mountain on the list? Do you want it to be?

Get clear about what type of life you want to live and what type of activities you want to be involved in. You don't have to be an athlete if you don't want to be. I guarantee you your list will include some type of movement, regardless, and that's all you need.

Setting the Stage

You may feel fear if you are not focused on being an athlete. You may assume that this will lead to being overweight or obese. Just remember that being an athlete is a choice, and it takes as much commitment as it would to be a lawyer or a doctor. It takes your focus and drive to be your best.

You wouldn't want a lawyer fighting your case who was only doing it because he thought he had to. Or a doctor performing your surgery who was only doing it because she thought she should. Just be who you are and don't apologize for what you are not.

Removing Negative Thoughts about Movement Increases Weight Loss Success

Movement is a way to live out your life fully. It is not a punishment for eating or gaining weight. When you make movement the means in which you shed weight, you are sabotaging your relationship with your ideal self.

Suddenly it doesn't matter that you just held warrior pose for five minutes because it didn't drop two pounds off your body. It begins to become negative and something you "have" to do instead of something you have the privilege to do. This is so unfair to movement and what it represents in our life. It's also unfair to you.

Your ideal self lives an ideal life – a life you dreamed of as a child and the one you picture in your clearest, most joyful moments. I guarantee this life involves movement. When you declare movement to be a "drag" or something you "hate" to do, you are telling your ideal self that you don't want to live your ideal life. When you don't appreciate movement for its own rewards and instead only find it worthwhile when you can see immediate physical results, then you are saying you don't enjoy or want the non-physical benefits movement brings.

You will not reach your goals of having an ideal body and an ideal life with those kinds of negative belief patterns. **If you are someone that "hates" exercise, then stop exercising immediately.** Ask yourself if you feel that way because you haven't found movement that you love yet, you have given it a negative meaning (weight loss), or your body truly just needs rest. **Then, make amends with movement and find what works for you and your body long term.**

Remember, you might not want to be an athlete. Being an athlete is not for everyone. When I was a trainer, people told me they wanted to hire me for better endurance. I would ask them if they were training for something, and they almost always said, “No.”

This told me that what they were really saying was that they believed extreme endurance was going to create some type of result in their life on an internal level. Some type of feeling or emotion, perhaps safety or confidence. They were trying to use movement to get physical results that they thought would lead to their ideal lives.

This is not how it works. You cannot use physical, external methods to create internal feelings. The results will always be temporary. You must “be” before you can “do” and “have.” The change has to come from the inside first.

So, ask yourself: What do you really want out of movement?

If you want endurance, you are going to have to do high-intensity activities. Make sure there are high-intensity activities you enjoy. If there are not, you need to ask yourself if endurance is really what you’re looking to achieve. What else might give you what you’re seeking? If you want strength, find a way to build it that you love. Also, ask yourself what you are looking to feel from having stronger muscles. Make sure you are filling this void on an internal level first.

Movement is a beautiful gift; don't ruin it by forcing yourself to be something you are not. If all you want to be is a person with some strength and endurance for everyday life, then this widens the options of movement.

My favorite movement is yoga. I absolutely love it. It makes my body and mind feel strong and calm in a way nothing else does. Would I be able to run a marathon from taking yoga three days a week? Probably not. But I don't want to run a marathon; I don't enjoy running enough to commit my life to it.

I am not an athlete; I am a coach, teacher, mentor, musician, and animal lover. And that is okay.

Who are you?

Homework Assignment #15
Connecting to My True Movement Desires

List the movements you will do when you are in your ideal body and why. Journal about who you are besides someone who moves. What makes you a unique individual? What makes you strong in non-physical ways?

Setting the Stage

As with the other exercises, be prepared for some fear that may arise as a result of being honest about your movement. What would happen if you took a break to rest? Would that make you fearful of weight gain? What about if you switched running to walking? Would you feel this was a waste of time?

Trust that whatever your body desires to do for movement is the right movement for you. Even if it's the wrong movement for someone else. Remember: What works for you is all that matters.

Listening to Your Body is the Best Way to Progress with Movement

There are going to be times when you have "yoga" on your calendar at 7 a.m., and you honestly need to sleep in. There are going to be other times when you skip yoga because you are allowing your autopilot to run, and it's not truly what you desire. Learning to distinguish between the two will help deepen your relationship with movement by ensuring you are giving yourself the love and care your body needs to thrive.

Telling the difference is simple in retrospect: If you skip the yoga, and you feel amazing, then it was the right decision. If you skip the yoga and greatly regret it, it was the wrong decision. Tuning in to how you felt before you made the decision to skip it will help you know to make the right decision in the future.

One important caveat: For communication to thrive between you and your body, you must exclude guilt. **Guilt is you feeling like you should do something because society, your spouse, or your parents said you should.**

Guilt is not an emotion given to us by Spirit. It's an emotion we learn from our society. Do not allow guilt to enter into your relationship with movement. It's toxic, and it will hinder your ability to listen to your intuition by ensuring you never give yourself the rest you need when you need it.

Look at the big picture. If you skip yoga three times in a row because you worked late and are tired, is that a big deal over the course of six months? Or a year? Or 10 years? Of course not.

You may fear that if you fall out of the pattern you may never return. If that's the truth, there is deeper work to do. If it's something you really love, why on earth would you never do it again?

Take a light approach with movement. Treat it like a hobby. You would never force yourself to go play guitar if you loved it. You would either feel like doing it or not. You wouldn't feel guilty if you didn't feel like playing guitar today, you would shrug it off and move on. Allow movement to exist in your life like any other activity.

And, even if it turns out that you wish you had gone to yoga that morning instead of sleeping in, don't be hard on yourself. You are learning. Now you know for the future that you really do want to go. As you practice listening to your body and honoring its needs, your intuition will get louder and louder, and you won't have to guess anymore about what you need. You will just have an inner knowing. You will automatically know when to move and when not to move.

Remember: For best results, move like you would if you were already in your ideal body.

Homework Assignment #16
No More "Shoulds"

Think about what you do each day. How much of what you do is what you want to do? How much is based on what you think you "should" do? Try to eliminate at least one "should" from your daily life each day. Focus on what your body is telling you it wants instead. Then, trust and follow your intuition. At the end of the day, write about how you feel.

Setting the Stage

Setting boundaries will be important in removing "shoulds" from your life. We can't do things for other people all the time if it sacrifices our own lives. To eliminate the "shoulds," you will have to say "No" to things. You potentially will have to disappoint someone. Grant yourself the room to do this.

Remember: You are not responsible for other people's expectations nor are you responsible for fulfilling their needs. Every person on the planet gets to choose his reaction to every situation so don't let fears over someone else's reaction make you tolerate "shoulds" that aren't serving you.

You have to do you ... always ... unapologetically.

Ideal Movement is Based on Intuition and Self-Love

Movement is not the “purge” to your “binge.” We don’t move so that we can eat food without gaining weight. We move because we can! Because we are alive and kicking, and it feels amazing.

Ideal movement – the kind of movement that increases our confidence and self-esteem and adds value to our ideal lives – is based on joy and self-love. It stems from our intuitions about what our bodies need and from the things that make us happy.

When you move, make sure you are honoring this tradition.

If you feel like slowly walking, great! If you feel like spin class, great! If you feel like slow dancing with your partner or spinning in circles with your child, great! It makes no difference what you do, it only matters that whatever it is feels loving and nurturing to **you**.

Don’t be fooled by the endless fitness articles that say you must work out for a certain amount of time and at a certain intensity. Though they say they’re geared toward weight loss, the truth is they are geared toward athletes.

If you don’t want to be an athlete, you don’t need to perform in athletic activities. Instead, you have the choice to move however you like for however long feels good to you. Consider movement as just another creative hobby. You wouldn’t trade in your guitar because you read painting was a “better” way to create, would you? Of course not! Do what feels best to you.

Homework Assignment #17
The Inspired Movement Challenge

Commit to only engaging in movements that bring you joy for an entire week. You might walk on Monday, dance on Tuesday, swim on Wednesday, and hit the gym on Thursday. You might play basketball every day or take a long walk every morning. The activities don't matter. What matters is that you take an inspired approach to movement and only move in a way that is loving and joyful for you. Notice how you feel before, during, and after the activities. Consider whether you are happier or feel healthier when you do what you love instead of when you do what you feel you "should" do.

Setting the Stage

Scratching your regular routine and only doing what feels good to you might make you anxious. You may worry that you'll gain weight during this time or lose muscle tone. Don't worry! Life always has a way of balancing itself out. There was a period of time when all I did was high-intensity cardio and weight lifting. Then all I wanted to do was yoga. For years! For years I did no cardio, just yoga. Then I felt like being in the gym again, just lifting weights. Then I felt like doing cardio again. I followed my intuition, and did what I felt like. And you know what? Through all of these changes my weight never fluctuated. Not even when I decided I needed a break and chose not to do any movement at all outside of daily living.

The only time my body fat increased was during a time when I wasn't doing any movement, yet I desperately wanted to. I wanted to take yoga and go to the gym, and I told myself I couldn't afford it. At that time, my body changed until I finally figured out a way to do what I loved to do. As soon as my movements were back in alignment with my body's desires, my body went back to normal.

Remember: There is no exact movement formula. Just do what feels good to you each day, and don't worry about your weight.

Movement Affirmations
(Pin these to your mirror, car, or anywhere they'll be seen regularly.)

My body loves to move.

It doesn't matter how hard I work or how much I sweat.

Any movement I do with full pleasure and presence is perfect for me today.

Movement is an opportunity to challenge my muscles and improve my health.

I move because I want and choose to move, not so I can eat.

Do

If you skipped straight to this chapter, go back and read the "being" section; trust me! Once you've read, understood, and actively engaged in the homework exercises in the "being" section, then turn back to this section and begin.

In this section I am going to give you some things to do. Let me be clear, my advice is not what you are most likely used to receiving.

For the most part, your entire weight loss journey is going to be focused on being. These steps are going to help you "just be" even easier. Here are some principles to keep in mind:

Everything discussed in the "doing" section should only be done when you desire to do it.

Don't force anything, and don't feel like you have to or should do anything either. Allow yourself to get to a place organically where you are excited to do these things.

If you feel extreme resistance for anything, get curious about it. Don't think that forcing yourself to try it is the answer.

Dig deep about why you feel such resistance and what you can do to get to a place where you have excitement to try something new.

Discover Your Core Falsities

In the first part of the book we talked about your subconscious mind and your internalized thoughts, beliefs, and patterns. Make sure you really understand how that works before you move forward into the next section of this book.

Remember: You will only be ready for the "doing" once you understand the "being."

This is because the first thing to do to lose weight is to make a decision that you are going to change your life. This means that from this point forward you will no longer live the same life. From this point forward you will only keep things that are serving you, and everything else will have to be let go.

Once you have made that decision and feel it all the way to your soul, get excited.

Because now the fun begins ...

It is time to become clear on what is false in your life or what is not serving you. Start a list of everything that you no longer want to experience. Be extremely honest about the things that do not align with your ideal life and body. Then, decide what gets to stay and what has to go.

Writing this list doesn't mean you have to throw everything out tomorrow. You can take baby steps. But, once you have this list, it’s time to become obnoxiously aware.

Change this big isn’t as easy as snapping your fingers. Your old patterns will continue to operate, even after you have decided that you don’t want them to do so. To move forward, you must notice old patterns, old thoughts, and old beliefs, and immediately correct them.

Thankfully, there are many ways to stop an old pattern.

You can begin doing something completely different, like blasting music. You could interrupt the pattern by screaming, “Stop It!” You could jump up and down and scream, or you could disprove the thought or belief. This could sound something like this:

Old Thought: “Okay, I have eaten 500 calories so far today so I have 1000 left.”

New Thought: “I just learned that calories don’t matter, and I no longer want to live my life as a slave to calories. There are tons of people who don’t count their calories and don’t have a weight problem so there is no need for me to live this way. I will no longer count my calories as of today."

This simple dialogue allows your old thought patterns to be retrained. It likely will take several times of having these types of conversations before you notice a change, but the more emotion you can pour in it the faster the old thoughts will disappear.

For those of you who have bigger things to remove from your life, such as a toxic relationship, you need to decide the best way to do this. Maybe you can simply cut off this person from affecting you negatively at first. You can master your ability not to allow their words to make you feel bad in any way. Completely distance yourself energetically, and pull your personal power back inside so that they have no power over you.

The first step to doing this is to recognize that you cannot change people. You can only control your own reactions to those people. For example, you may have a spouse who calls you fat. In your old way of thinking you might have thought: "My spouse tells me I am fat, therefore my spouse is mean and I feel bad and pressured to lose weight." Then, you might tell your spouse to quit calling you fat, commit to working out even more or eating even less, and then berate yourself when you fail to measure up to your impossibly high expectations.

The new you – the one living his or her ideal life – doesn't do that. Instead, the new you chooses to approach the situation from a place of power by claiming responsibility for the situation and your reactions to that situation.

You are responsible for being in the relationship with your spouse. You are responsible for feeling and responding sensitively to someone's comments about your weight. You are responsible for your feelings of external pressure and failure. You have chosen all of these things, whether you like them or not.

Knowing this doesn't mean you blame yourself. Instead, it empowers you to make new choices and to design the life you want, one with situations that make you happy instead of upset.

This mindset is incredibly freeing and empowering. You are not at anyone's mercy. If you don't like someone's behavior, you can leave the situation or change your reaction to it so that it no longer affects you negatively. Instead of feeling pressured and upset when your spouse calls you fat, you can choose not to take it personally. You know you are living your ideal life and your ideal body is emerging. You are on your way. If someone, even your spouse, says something about you, the new you knows it is about them, not you.

You also can do this type of exercise with a toxic work environment. If you are not able to simply quit right away, begin removing yourself energetically from the toxicity. Begin telling yourself that you are going to be the best version of yourself while you are there and block anything that gets in the way. You can make an internal shift, energetically, and get results even before you are ready to leave a toxic situation. You are that powerful.

TIP: When you shift how you feel, your external world will shift as well.

If this feels right, then start here. If it doesn't, or if you know that you are not able to create an effective boundary, then come up with a plan for removing yourself from the situation altogether. Just remember that your environment will influence your results.

If I could bring you to my house and sit you in front of me for 60 days in a row, not allowing you to go back into your old environment, then you would drop the weight instantly because you would know you are safe and protected energetically. Of course, I can't do that, which means you have to do it for yourself.

You will not be able to take your old self – your old environment, thoughts, beliefs, and patterns – into your new way of living. It is impossible. To live a new life, in a new body, you must be a new you. You will have to do your best to create this type of energetic sanctuary for yourself by creating the necessary boundaries to get the results you desire. It is the only way to eliminate what isn't serving you from your life for good.

You may notice as you begin this transformation that old patterns continue to creep in. Do not judge or berate yourself for this. Be patient with the new you. Remember: The new patterns and beliefs you desire to embody are just that – new. They are fresh and fragile. They are also easily forgotten.

For example, you may finish this book and decide to discuss your next steps with your spouse. You may be super excited and amped up about making these changes, and expecting supportive dialogue with a hint of respect for your newfound mindset. But, instead of giving you the boost you wanted, your spouse does the complete opposite.

“Yeah right, good luck with that,” he or she says. “You can’t lose weight unless you eat less and move more.”

And there it is. All that excitement, gone in less than 10 seconds.

Likely this will happen with someone. People around you will attempt to inform you of their beliefs, their experiences. They will try to prove you wrong.

Don’t let this get to you. Their actions aren’t malicious. They are human, and as humans they find it difficult to change long-held beliefs. While you are finally in the “right moment” of your life to be receptive to a new way of being, others require their own right moments. Your actions are unrelated to their timing.

This is why it’s so important in the beginning part of this journey that you allow yourself time to embody these principles. You will be faced with experiences every single day that could cause you to run back to your old ways of thinking, your old ways of being, for safety. Some days, it will feel easier and more comfortable to abort this mission and return to old dieting methods.

The only way to push through this phase is to remind yourself of the discoveries you made in the first part of this journey. Now that you know the core falsities you carried with you for so long, you will want to revisit them often. You will want to remind yourself that they are not you, that you desire another way. You will also want to remind yourself that the people around you, even those you love, may not understand the journey you've undertaken, and that it's okay.

You don't have to carry your falsities in your back pocket (although you can), you just need to recognize them when they creep back in to your life (which absolutely they will try to do). This will happen most likely during moments of mindlessness, when you let the everyday moments of life switch you to autopilot. Watching TV, eating, and driving a car are common moments of such inattention.

During these everyday actions, you act in automatic ways. Along with these automatic behaviors come automatic thoughts, beliefs, and patterns. Until you have completely mastered your new set of thoughts, beliefs, and patterns, this is where your old ways of being will try hardest to reclaim you. To keep moving steadily toward your goals, these are the moments when you will want to be especially present and bring an extra sense of consciousness to your tasks.

If you are driving, you might try listening to books or empowering speakers – things that keep you mentally engaged. If you are eating, you will want to practice slow mindful eating during which you focus all of your attention on the satisfaction and pleasure you are getting from the experience. If you are watching TV, try watching shows that make you feel empowered, such as "What Not to Wear," which emphasizes the importance of a healthy body image. (For now, avoid shows that bring up your insecurities, shows in which you see perfect bodies and shallow living, for instance.)

By making these changes, you are not eliminating your autopilot entirely. Nor should you. That's not the goal. The goal is to give yourself enough time to become so fully your ideal self that those moments begin to reinforce your new ways of being, instead of the old.

In the beginning, when you are working hard to maintain these fragile new thoughts, patterns, and beliefs, you also may want to set yourself up for success by creating new experiences around these more habitual experiences. Eat in new places. Take new routes to familiar destinations. Practice a new hobby instead of watching TV or playing video games or surfing the web. Any or all of these things will keep you actively engaged and prevent your autopilot from derailing your progress.

Once you've grown stronger in your new way of being, you still will want to check in with your body and your intuition frequently to watch for moments when you begin slipping into a way of living that doesn't serve your ideal self. Watch for moments when your muscles tense up or your belly does a flip-flop. Watch for times when you feel restless and are wiggling and fretting in your chair, anxiously unable to sit still. Feelings like these are communications from your body that it doesn't like whatever is going on at that moment. These are your body's signals that something is off.

Some of you may feel a sense of low energy or depression. This is also a signal of something being off. Some of you may feel an overall feeling of irritability or a general need to escape. Everyone is different and your body's unique signals will be different than anyone else's, but the message is always the same: Something is wrong; something needs to be changed.

When these signals are ignored for days, months, or years, the body will send louder and louder signals. Eventually weight gain and physical illness will set in. As long as you stay present, though, and continue to make the changes described in the "being" section of this book, the inevitable moments of relapse will be temporary and will have zero effect on your body and weight. By reminding you of what doesn't serve you, they even can ultimately bring you closer to what does.

Find Out What Fuels You

Now that you have removed what is not serving you from your life, it's time to add more of what is. Most people I've talked to admit they don't have a whole lot of hobbies or fun in their lives. Instead, they fill their days with work, being a parent, and doing things for other people. Once evening rolls around, they're exhausted, and the only thing they can think of to do is to grab a snack and turn on the TV.

There is nothing wrong with relaxing and enjoying food and entertainment, but make sure you are filling your days and nights with activities and foods that truly fulfill you.

TIP: The next time you sit down in front of the TV, ask yourself, "Is this really what I want to be doing or is it what I am settling to do?"

If you find you're settling, but can't think of anything else to do, get creative. Begin trying new things. Ask your friends what hobbies they participate in and join them. Look at your local community college for some inexpensive classes to try. Take this time to discover your passion – a reason to live besides your career, your relationships, and your kids. Ask yourself, "If all of that were to go away, who would I be?" What would you want your life to look like?

Consider, for example, an obligation-free weekend. Your spouse takes the kids away on a trip. Your house is completely clean. The laundry is all washed, folded, and hung. There are no work deadlines or unfinished projects hanging over your head. Your time is completely your own.

What do you do?

If your answer involves some kind of electronics – Internet, TV, DVD players, or video games – eliminate them. Imagine the power goes out or the devices are all malfunctioning. What do you do then?

What if the weekend turns into a week? Two weeks? A month? What do you do?

The point of finding your passion/s is that you'll never again have to wonder what you'd do in the above scenario. You'll know. And, you'll be thrilled to have the time, the space, and the quiet to just be you, by yourself, with yourself.

This is your goal.

In order to create the most magnificent life for yourself, you have to get to the point where you can be happy just being you. Where you have passion for yourself and your life. Once you get there, your body will thrive and blossom from the joyful and fulfilled life you're living. Any issues with your weight will be gone.

Transformation happens as a result of living your best life. It happens when we are present and thriving. When we are living each moment with presence. When we're living our ideal lives, our bodies no longer need the heaviness. They no longer need protective layers and false beliefs. Instead, they can finally reveal the ideal body inside.

TIP: Have as much fun as possible!

Allow your days to fly by, not because you are constantly staying busy, but because you are too busy living life to the fullest. Allow your desire to lose weight to push you to action. Allow the motivation to have your ideal body to be strong enough that you are willing to get uncomfortable and try new things. Give your life so much meaning that your body has no choice but to transform to give you the ability to do all the fun, meaningful things you so desire to do.

Meditate

Most people are constantly doing. Running from one thing to the next, barely stopping to breathe. Then, they either do high-intensity exercise, continuing the constant state of doing, or they plop down on the couch, exhausted from knowing they have to do it all again tomorrow. They may turn on the TV, in an effort to relax and "do nothing," but TV isn't really relaxing because it isn't an active process. Watching TV is something that happens to you, it isn't something you do.

To really thrive in your ideal life, you need to practice intentional "not doing." Meditation is a great method of achieving this.

Meditation enables you to move intentionally from doing back into being, thereby increasing your intuition and helping you connect with your ideal self. It helps you recharge and rejuvenate. It also helps you de-stress, which is essential for maintaining your ideal life and body.

TIP: Slow down and take a timeout from life.

Our society discourages quiet time and relaxation so I understand that many of you will find it challenging to do absolutely nothing. Some of you may even find the idea torturous. But, if you try it, you'll likely be amazed at how it makes you feel.

Start small, perhaps with guided meditations, to begin to learn how to quiet your mind and focus on something other than the busyness of your day. Eventually, you'll want to work on slowing down your breath, but for now just notice it. Notice each inhalation and each exhalation. Try to keep your body still and your mind focused on the steady in and out.

At first, you may experience a lot going on as you sit quietly. Your mind may race with thoughts. You might find yourself tapping your feet or opening your eyes constantly. You may be unable to keep still without shifting your position for more than a few seconds at a time. This is okay. In fact, it is expected. You'll still get results – even with all of that going on – because it is still less "doing" than you experience in your everyday moments.

Once you're able to sit quietly and mindfully attend your breath for five to 10 minutes at a time, try consciously altering the depth and speed of each breath until you are breathing deeply in and deeply out at a slow, steady pace.

Most of us spend the day breathing shallowly and quickly. This triggers our sympathetic nervous system (our fight-or-flight response), and floods our bodies with stress hormones. These hormones tell our bodies we are in danger, which alters our digestion and metabolic functions. Instead of digesting and metabolizing food or burning fat, our bodies think they have to store the nutrients for later.

Slow, long, deliberate breathing, on the other hand, triggers the parasympathetic nervous system, which triggers a relaxation response. This system tells our bodies to relax. It says, "Go ahead and burn fat, digest food; you're fine. No bears coming toward us today. No need to run."

By slowing, deepening, and lengthening our breathing in meditation, we bring both our emotional and our physical selves into balance. This not only saves our sanity, but it aids weight loss efforts. The more time you spend engaging the parasympathetic nervous system, the more you are allowing your body to perform optimally and the easier time your body will have releasing excess weight.

I suggest meditating right before bed or first thing in the morning for about 10 to 15 minutes. If this doesn't work for you, however, don't worry. The important thing is not when you do it or how long you do it, it is that you make meditation a regular part of your life, even if that means you simply sit and focus on your breathing for five minutes on your lunch hour. You can also try meditating for just a couple of minutes anytime you feel overwhelmed or sleepy. You'll be surprised at how much better you feel!

Dive Into Self Care

We all know that in order to have a healthy, happy body we need to take care of ourselves. Yet, we've all had periods of time in which we ate foods that weren't good for us, neglected our bodies' needs for movement and relaxation, and simply ignored the communications our bodies were sending. Often, at the same time, we complained that we didn't feel good or that we didn't like the way we looked (maybe both). We also seemed unable to put two and two together and realize that the neglect we were showing our bodies was causing all our problems.

What gives? How can we be the smart, intelligent humans that we are and yet miss such an important and seemingly simple connection?

In order to have a desire to take care of ourselves, we must actually believe that we are worth being taken care of.

A negative self-image can make it nearly impossible to bridge the gap between knowing it's important to take care of ourselves and actually doing it. Hopefully, the first section of this book helped you identify and toss out the false beliefs and negative thought patterns that weren't serving you. Hopefully, you have made tremendous gains in your self-esteem and are exhibiting renewed and increased self-love every day. Hopefully, you're no longer berating yourself for not adhering to someone else's expectations of you. It's likely though, especially early on in the journey to your ideal life, that you may need to be reminded of your worth every now and again.

So, do it. Remind yourself day by day, hour by hour if necessary, that you are worthy. That you have value. That you are loveable and loved. Right now, exactly as you are.

Kick out any old thoughts or beliefs that try to sneak in and tell you otherwise. Remember that they are false, that they stem from thoughts and beliefs that were given to you by someone else and that they are not your own. Remember that you do not have to believe them. Remember that you **don't** believe them.

Tell yourself, again and again and again, that you are absolutely worthy of whatever you desire. Write "I am worthy" on post-it notes and stick them all over your house, if it makes you feel better. Send yourself emails with "You are worthy" in the subject line. Play feel-good songs very loudly while singing at the top of your lungs. Whatever works for you.

Only once you believe you are worthy of love, will you show yourself love. And, self-love must come before self-care, because we take care of the things we love. You can't trick your body into thinking you love it in order to get the results you desire, however. Your body isn't easily fooled. You must show it authentic love before it will show you results.

So how do you get there?

You love your body by making peace with where you are and admitting that your body didn't do "this" to you, it's just where you are.

If you and a friend got in a fight and you decided the relationship was worth saving, what would you do? You might start by recognizing how you carry responsibility for what happened between you and your friend. Then, you might forgive the other person for things they did or said in order to move forward with peace. Lastly, you would set up a communication with that person to express your feelings and move forward together with love.

Apply this same process to your body.

Recognize the negative things you've done to your body. Forgive your body for not being perfect. Accept that it is doing the best it can with what you've given it over the years. Then, listen to it. Slow down when your body tells you it needs a break. Stop eating when it says it is full. Eat when it says it is hungry. Move in the way it wants when it needs movement.

Building this relationship with your body will allow your love for you to grow. As it does, your desire to take care of yourself also will grow. Once you believe you are worthy of all that you desire and you've created a healthy and loving relationship with your body, then you are ready to introduce **gentle** self-care habits into your life.

TIP: Self-care never involves force.

It would be impossible for me to tell you exactly what to do to take care of your body. Everyone is different, and everyone needs different things. It's your job to listen to what your body needs and to respect those needs.

If your body is asking for rest, rest.

If it's asking for water, give it water.

If it's asking for food, stop everything and give it food.

If it's asking for more movement, start moving.

If it's asking for a hot bath, take a hot bath.

If it's asking for a massage, have one, whether it's at a fancy spa, a trade with a friend, or a self-massage.

If your skin is asking for TLC, give it what it needs, with a slow and thorough exfoliation or a special face treatment or by applying natural oils.

If your hands, feet, or any part of your body is asking for more oxygen, give them the slow stretches they need to breathe.

You're getting these signals every single day. The more you listen for them, the louder they get.

Check in with your habits. If you are abusing caffeine, sugar, cigarettes, drugs, alcohol, or anything else in excess, take a moment to assess the situation. What are these things doing for you? How are they working with your body? How can you make different choices with your body in mind? You may need more help in these areas than this book can provide, and that's perfectly okay. Just begin to set up steps to help you achieve the highest level of self-care possible.

Start where you are. This journey is a marathon, not a sprint. Start with self-worth and accept that you may be there for a while. Enjoy that part of the journey. When you're ready, begin practicing self-love. Watch as how you care for yourself begins to transform.

TIP: The more patient and present you can be with the process, the more fun you will have.

When we get too attached to the end result, we make it impossible to enjoy the present moment, and we make the journey feel forced and rushed. There are incredible lessons for you to learn right here, right now. Stay here for as long as you need to stay here. Allow your life to unfold at a pace that isn't determined by you. This level of trust and freedom will create a lighter life, which is what you truly desire anyway, isn't it?

Eat Consciously

Earlier in this book, you learned how important it is to slow down at mealtimes, remove stress around food, and listen to your body's messages about what it wants and needs. Now, it's time to put all that into practice by eating consciously.

Remember: To get your ideal body, you have to eat like you already have your ideal body. Conscious eating is a fun, relaxing way to do that.

Before each meal, make sure you set the stage for a healthy eating experience by choosing high quality food. It's important to choose nutritious, minimally processed foods whenever possible, so that you can access your highest level of self-care and health. This doesn't mean you can't enjoy junk food when you desire, but it does mean you stop to assess the quality of the foods you eat, especially the foods you eat most often.

Once you sit down to eat, stay present and calm. Remind yourself that whatever food you're eating should nourish you, physically and emotionally. If you feel stressed or tense or if you begin to think negative thoughts about food, stop right away and reassess the situation. Try meditating for a few moments to allow your new way of being to overcome any old thought patterns and beliefs that may be bothering you. If you are still feeling bothered or anxious, consider what your body is telling you. Are the foods you are about to eat what your body wants and needs? If so, relax, dig in, and enjoy! If not, consider what your body might prefer instead.

During the meal, practice active awareness. Wake up at the plate, and stay awake until the meal is over. Notice your physical and emotional reactions to the food you eat. Do you like it? Does it satisfy you? Notice also when you are hungry and when you are full, and stop when your body tells you to stop. For those of you who struggle with overeating, this will be the most important step for you to master. Staying relaxed throughout the meal will help.

The easiest way to relax and slow down during your meals is to practice deep breathing as you eat. Take a bite, then take a deep breath. Take a bite, then take a deep breath. The act of slow, conscious breathing allows your body to relax and enjoy the food more deeply.

Pay close attention to whether you are getting pleasure from your meal. In a society that views food as little more than fuel, it's often challenging to imagine that pleasure is an important component of why we eat. Without it, however, your brain won't send the signals that tell you you're full, and you'll keep eating more and more food until you obtain the satisfaction you truly desire. If you notice that whatever you're eating isn't fulfilling your emotional needs, stop eating immediately. Then, listen closely to your body until you figure out what will give you the pleasure you're seeking. Once you know the answer, respond to your body with love and appreciation by giving it what it wants.

Once you've reached satiety, the meal is over, but the act of conscious eating is not. Maintain awareness of how you feel over the next one to 24 hours. Notice whether you feel lighter or heavier as the day progresses. Consider what that means for your body and your future food choices.

By eating consciously, you are treating your body with the love and respect it deserves – exactly what it needs to transform into the ideal version of itself. Practice conscious eating at every meal, and you'll be amazed at how quickly your body transforms.

Value Health

We all have a value system. Some of us value family and friends. Some value money and career. Others value health. Most of us value a combination of these things.

If you want to live inside your ideal body, you must prioritize health in the list of things you value.

A person who values money over health will go into a grocery store and choose the cheapest bread they can find. It won't matter what the ingredients are, or how healthy it is. They only care that it's the cheapest. A person who values health more than money will do the opposite. He will stand in the aisle, reading each bread's label, until he finds the one he believes is the healthiest. That's the one he'll choose to buy.

These are exaggerated examples, of course (most of us read labels *and* price tags to make a decision that balances both), but the comparison is meant to show one thing: Your value system dictates the decisions you make on a day-to-day basis. So, decide, right now, that you place a premier value on health. Then, have fun!

Get creative in the kitchen. Healthy food can be incredibly delicious. Try new ingredients you have never cooked with or a new genre of food. Take a cooking class or learn about wine pairing. Amp up your dinner first. Grab some cookbooks, find some recipes that are calling to you, and plan out your week. (Cookbooks like "French Women Don't Get Fat," with simple ingredients and clean recipes, may be easiest for beginner cooks.) Experiment with plating your food and setting the table.

TIP: Use a Crockpot to reduce time spent in the kitchen, and shop at local, healthy grocery stores and farmers' markets to reduce your costs and automatically surround yourself with healthier ingredients.

The more fun you can have with your food, the more you will start to see the value in experiencing health *through* your food. And the more you do that, the easier it will be to stick to your new routines. Approach exercise in the same way. The more fun you can have with your exercise, the more you will start to see the value in experiencing health *through* your exercise.

Notice how amazing your body feels when you move it. Notice how it feels when you don't move it. Listen to the little voice inside that tells you it wants to move.

TIP: When you value health, you will naturally be drawn to move simply for the health benefits.

When you exercise for health reasons there are no rules. There are no "have-tos." It no longer matters if you sweated through a high-intensity workout or simply lied on the floor in a yoga class. Any movement that you enjoy and your body wants is great for your health.

Experiment with exercise just like with food. Join a gym that has lots of classes and try them all. Get outside of your comfort zone and try belly dancing or pole dancing or a new sport. Don't worry about making a "wrong" decision. There are no wrong decisions when you're placing a high value on health and following your intuition.

Tip: When you value health above all else, you can't make changes in your food and exercise and fail.

As long as what you are doing allows your body to feel better, you're succeeding.

Have

We are finally here. You have learned how to change who you are being. You have learned what to do to help you achieve your goals, and now it's time to have the body and life you desire. So what's next?

Full surrender and trust.

That is the last piece of the puzzle.

Many people will want to read this book, and then have the information magically flow into their bodies and transform immediately. They want the list that they can check off and say, "I did these things so now I can have what I want."

That isn't how it works.

There isn't a formula that you can follow that will give you your ideal body. (Remember the "calories in versus calories out" rule?) You cannot force or control your way into it, either. Instead, you have to trust: trust that the process is working and that you are already in your ideal body – right here, right now.

It's covered in layers of old thoughts, beliefs, and patterns.

It's covered with old information that isn't serving you.

It's covered in baggage and protection.

It's covered in fear, worry, and doubt.

But, it's there.

Underneath all that weight, your ideal body is waiting, ready to be revealed.

So start peeling the layers and trust in the process. You are doing exactly what you need to be doing right now. Believe in yourself. Believe in the process. Trust your body.

When you begin to feel afraid that the weight may not come off and you need to control something (and this will happen, do not beat yourself up for it!) breathe into your fear and realign your thoughts in a positive manner.

Check into your need to control and journal about it. Meditate on trust and surrender. Notice that the more you let go of control, the more uncomfortable you may feel. Know that eventually you will adjust, and you will enjoy the freedom of having no rules for your body and weight.

Remember: There is nothing for you to consciously control about your body. Your subconscious is taking care of it. Your only job is to live your most incredible life. Go out there and live it!

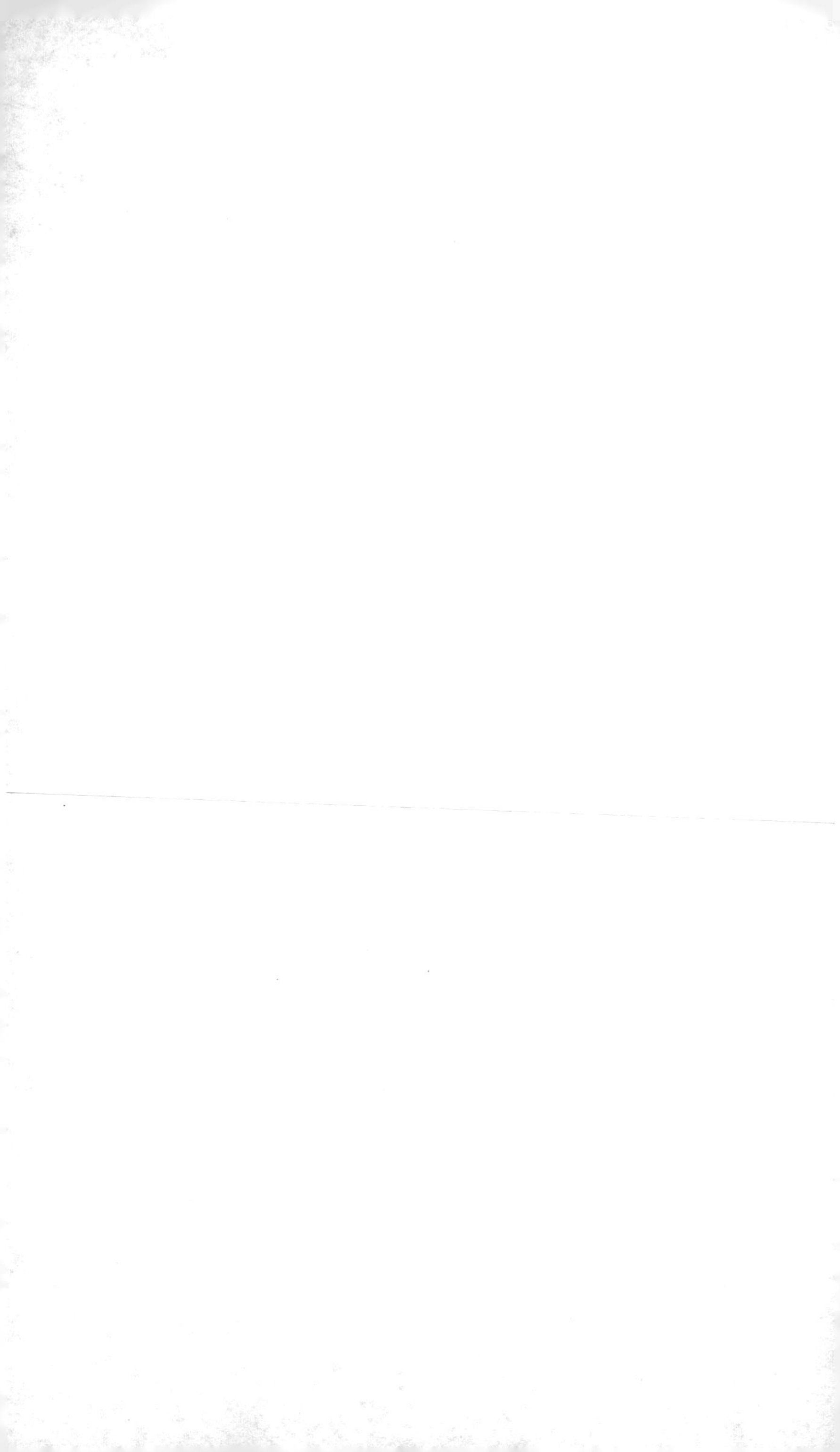

Bonus: How to Use Self-Hypnosis

One of my favorite ways to achieve powerful change is through self-hypnosis. This book provided ideas on how to consciously change your thoughts, beliefs, and patterns. Self-hypnosis adds an additional element by enabling you to speak directly to your subconscious beliefs and patterns without your conscious mind arguing or negating the positive suggestions. By incorporating self-hypnosis into your daily life, you can create change easily and effortlessly.

Self-hypnosis achieves results similar to meditation, but it carries with it the explicit goal of altering the underlying subconscious patterns and beliefs that created the issue you are addressing.

For DIY self-hypnosis audios, you can use the recording option on your phone or on your computer to create personalized hypnoses using the following scripts. Feel free to add your own hypnotic suggestions as well. If you have audio editing software, you can add music. Otherwise, feel free to play relaxing music on another device as you listen to your own voice recording.

Once you have recorded your hypnoses, find a quiet place where you can relax and close your eyes. It's crucial to the success of these recordings that you are completely relaxed. Quiet your mind, release any tension in your muscles, and focus on your breath.

For some of you, entering a state conducive to self-hypnosis may take time. I, too, am someone with a busy mind so I often will listen to 30-45 minutes of guided meditation before I listen to my hypnosis. You may not have that amount of time to spend on meditation, and that's okay. Find a balance that works for you.

(A great place to find free guided meditations is from Meditation Oasis. This is a free podcast on iTunes that has tons of fantastic meditations.)

At first, upon completion of the hypnosis, you may be unsure if you were "under" or if you had merely fallen asleep. Pay attention to *when* you come back into awareness. If you come back into awareness as the recording is telling you to do so, there is a good chance you did not fall asleep. If you wake up and the recording is off, and you're not sure when it went off, you may have fallen asleep. But, that's fine too. I truly believe the recording is still being heard when we fall asleep. So let go, and allow your body to tell you what it needs. (It may be sleep!)

The more you practice self-hypnosis, the faster changes in

your life will occur. For perspective: think about how often you hear negative suggestions, both the negative thoughts that run through your mind and the ones that come from others. Even by simply being in a public space, you could hear hundreds of potentially negative things that could negate the positive beliefs I explained in this book.

Therefore, in order for these messages to become a permanent part of your life, you will need to experience them repeatedly. Listen to at least one of these hypnoses every day, and you will notice positive change in your life. It may not be obvious at first; sometimes it initially goes almost unnoticed. But, one day, you will become aware that you haven't overeaten in a week or that you haven't been obsessing over your exercise or that you haven't been critical of your body. This is how you will know self-hypnosis is working.

I often practice right when I wake up (with a backup alarm in case I fall back asleep) or right before bed. These are times when we are naturally more relaxed, which makes it easier to let go of conscious control and allow change to happen on the subconscious level.

Below is an Intro and an Outro that can be recorded for each session, followed by several example scripts of what can be recorded in the middle of each session.

Intro: This will help you come into a state of relaxation and be open and receptive to the self-hypnosis suggestions.

Take a deep breath, and begin to relax completely. Let go of your busy day, your busy thoughts.

You have no other place to be, absolutely nothing to do.

Begin by feeling your toes relax completely, releasing any tension in the process.

Then, move up to your ankle and the bottom half of your leg. Notice as they, too, relax completely.

Now, turn your attention to the top of your leg, through the pelvis and all the way into your hips. Feel that part of your body begin to relax as well.

As you move through your belly and low back, and up through your chest and shoulders, feel your body relax completely with each breath.

Your neck releases its tension, and your head begins to drop. Your jaw relaxes, your tongue comes off the roof of your mouth, and your forehead completely lets go of all of its tension.

Moving up to the crown of your head, feel your entire body relax. Bring your inner gaze to your third eye center, in between your eyebrows, in your mind's eye.

Remember you are safe, and feel a wave of love and comfort wash over you.

Now feeling so relaxed, begin to notice a set of stairs directly in front of you. You become aware that this set of stairs will lead you into a deep, deep state of hypnosis where you will feel better than you have ever felt before.

You know with certainty that as you walk down each step, you will feel more and more relaxed and only good things will come of this state of relaxation.

You take the first step down the staircase, feeling so safe and so relaxed.

You take the second and third steps down into deep, deep hypnosis.

Four, Five, and Six, feeling the relaxation that comes from each step.

Seven, Eight … so so relaxed.

Nine and Ten. You now feel more relaxed than you ever have felt before.

You are open and ready to receive the suggestions you are about to hear.

Outro: This goes at the end of each recording to bring you back into wakeful awareness.

You now begin to notice a set of stairs in the distance. You begin to walk toward the staircase feeling so wonderful, light, and free.

As you walk up each step, you know you will begin to come back into the room with full awareness.

You are now fully aware and awake and feel wonderful. You are your best self.

Scripts

Being the Person Who Gets Results Script

You are ready to become someone who gets the results you desire in life. You know that absolutely anything is possible in this limitless world, and you choose to believe only the thoughts and beliefs that are in alignment with where you want to go.

You are worthy of everything that you desire, and you are completely loved.

You are completely safe and secure and free to have anything you desire.

You know exactly how to take care of yourself and achieve all of your goals and desires, and you do so with attentive self-care and self-love.

You are a person who spends time enjoying the activities that matter most to you, someone with unbounded energy and enthusiasm.

You are happy with your body and your life. You place a high value on self-care, self-love, and your overall health.

You feel confident as you go after what you want, and you allow what you desire to come to you. You let go of your need for the path to be hard or full of struggles. You are happy for rewards to come easily and effortlessly. You let go of the necessity of hard work in order to easily and effortlessly have what you desire.

<Add any additional hypnotic suggestions you like here>

Being One with Your Body Script

You are open and ready to accept and love your body as it is today. You know with certainty that loving and accepting your body is the path to having all that you desire.

As you find more love and acceptance, and let go of fear, your body is becoming lighter and lighter more and more every day.

You operate with the basic understanding that your body already knows how to be ideal for you. You trust that your body will guide you to what you desire each and every day without fear.

You know, now, how incredible your body is, and you want to work with it to feel lighter today.

You recognize the power of love and acceptance and feel this becoming your reality today, now.

As you feel lighter and lighter, with ease you find more confidence, contentment, and understanding for who you are and what your body is now.

You let go of the body needing to be perfect and realize your body is simply a vessel, not something to provide emotions or meet your needs. You know how to meet your own needs regardless of the circumstances of your body.

<Add any additional hypnotic suggestions you like here>

Being One with Food Script

You find yourself easily and effortlessly eating slowly. You are relaxed as you digest your food and your body feels this level of awareness through relaxation.

You feel your metabolism becoming quick and efficient as you enjoy all the foods your body is asking for.

You prefer to sit at the table with presence and enjoy every bite of your food, so much that you find yourself being satisfied with less. You notice you can leave a bite of food on your plate without the need to eat it.

You feel relaxed as you eat your food and your body feels the lightness from this. Food gives you pleasure, and you only eat it when you are hungry and open to receiving this pleasure.

You easily notice when you feel the urge to eat outside of hunger, and you effortlessly choose what you desire to do instead. You feel your emotions and know with certainty that food is not the healer of your emotions.

You love food and trust yourself and your appetite. You crave high quality food that fills you up, gives you nourishment, and leaves you satisfied and fulfilled. You are sensationally aware of how poorly low quality food tastes and feels in your body.

You give yourself extreme self-love and self-care through the foods you choose, with full love and appreciation.

<Add any additional hypnotic suggestions you like here>

Being One with Movement Script

You love to move your body. Your body feels better when it's moving regularly. You feel your body gaining strength and endurance as it moves freely in your daily activities.

You operate with an understanding that your body always chooses to move when it has the energy to do so, and you find a balance between work, play, and rest so that your energy is full.

You find excitement in participating in activities that require you to challenge and move your body. You are open to trying new activities to see if they are fun and fulfilling for you.

You know that everyone is paying attention to their own selves as you move. You release the need to look a certain way as you move and accept that everyone starts somewhere.

You love to have full presence and awareness while you move your body, and you love the feeling of your muscles working together to complete an activity. You prefer to have presence in the moment rather than to distract yourself.

You know exactly when your body needs rest and when it needs movement and honor whatever your body is asking for.

You allow movement to be a way to increase your health, increase your strength, and increase your endurance. You ask nothing else of it. You allow movement to be free and fun.

<Add any additional hypnotic suggestions you like here>

About Michelle Hastie

Michelle Hastie is the author of "The Weight Loss Shift: Be More, Weigh Less" and a contributor to the women's studies bestseller, "Women Will Save the World." A weight loss coach, Michelle helps chronic dieters surrender to their body wisdom in order to lose weight permanently. Using a blend of science, psychology, and spirituality, Michelle helps people live incredible lives in bodies they love! She has a background in personal training, food psychology, neuro-linguistic programming, and yoga and has been featured in SHAPE magazine over a dozen times for her life changing gift of transforming lives, one body at a time. She is available for virtual coaching at www.totalbodyhealthsolutions.com.

About Absolute Love Publishing

Absolute Love Publishing is an independent book publisher devoted to creating and publishing projects that promote goodness in the world.

We have published internationally renowned and Billboard-topping musicians, Olympic athletes, prominent media professionals and authors, inspirational and visionary figures, innovative change-makers, spiritual leaders, and others. Absolute Love Publishing is located in Austin, Texas, USA. It owns min-e-book.com and the trademark, min-e-book™. A min-e-book™ is a shorter-style e-book designed for a quick read.

Absolute Love Publishing is also home to the imprint Spirited Press, an independent (assisted self-publishing) platform that assists writers in sharing their own messages with the world through a la carte book editing, marketing, and publishing services.

www.AbsoluteLovePublishing.com
www.min-e-book.com
www.SpiritedPress.com
www.WomenWillSavetheWorld.com
http://blog.absolutelovepublishing.com/
www.Shop.AbsoluteLovePublishing.com
Facebook: www.facebook.com/Absolute.Love.Publishing
Pinterest: www.pinterest.com/AbsoluteLovePub/
Twitter: www.twitter.com/AbsoluteLovePub

Books by Absolute Love Publishing

Adventures of a Lightworker: Dead End Date

"Dead End Date" is the first book in a metaphysical series about a woman's crusade to teach the world about love, one mystery and personal hang-up at a time. In a Bridget Jones meets New Age-style, "Dead End Date" introduces readers to Faith, a young woman whose dating disasters and personal angst have separated her from the reason she's on Earth. When she receives the shocking news that she is a lightworker and has one year to fulfill her life purpose, Faith embarks on her mission with zeal, tackling problems big and small – including the death of her blind date. Working with angels and psychic abilities and even the murder victim himself, Faith dives headfirst into a personal journey that will transform all those around her and, eventually, all those around the world.

Finding Happiness with Migraines: a Do It Yourself Guide by Sarah Hackley, a min-e-book™

Do you have monthly, weekly, or even daily migraines? Do you feel lonely or isolated, or like you are constantly worrying about the next impending migraine? Is the weight of living with migraines dampening your enjoyment of the "now"? Experience the happiness you crave with "Finding Happiness with Migraines: a Do It Yourself Guide," a min-e-book™ by Sarah Hackley. Discover how you can take charge of your body, your mind, your emotions, and your health by practicing simple, achievable steps that create a daily life filled with more joy, appreciation, and confidence. Sarah's Five Steps to Finding Happiness with

Migraines provide an actionable path to a new, happier way of living with migraines. A few of the tools you'll learn: which yoga poses can help with a migraine attack, why you should throw away your daily migraine journal, how do-it-yourself therapy can create positive change, and techniques to connect with your body and intuition.

Love Like God: Embracing Unconditional Love

In this groundbreaking compilation, well-known individuals from across the globe share stories of how they learned to release the conditions that block absolute love. Along with the insights of bestselling author Caroline A. Shearer, readers will be reminded of their natural state of love and will begin to envision a world without fear or judgement or pain. Along with Shearer's reflections and affirmations, experts, musicians, authors, professional athletes, and others shed light on the universal experiences of journeying the path of unconditional love.

Love Like God Companion Book

You've read the love-expanding essays from the luminaries of "Love Like God." Now, take your love steps further with the "Love Like God Companion Book." The Companion provides a positive, actionable pathway into a state of absolute love, enabling readers to further open their hearts at a pace that matches their experiences. This book features an expanded introduction, the Thoughts and Affirmations from "Love Like God," plus all new "Love in Action Steps."

Raise Your Financial Vibration: Tips and Tools to Embrace Your Infinite Spiritual Abundance, a min-e-book™

Are you ready to release the mind dramas that hold you back from your infinite spiritual abundance? Are you ready for a high-frequency financial life? Allow, embrace, and enjoy your infinite spiritual abundance and financial wealth today! Absolute Love Publishing Creator Caroline A. Shearer explores simple steps and shifts in mindset that will help you receive the abundance you desire in "Raise Your Financial Vibration: Tips and Tools to Embrace Your Infinite Spiritual Abundance," a min-e-book™. Learn how to release blocks to financial abundance, create thought patterns that will help you achieve a more desirable financial reality, and fully step into an abundant lifestyle by discovering the art of *being* abundant.

Raise Your Verbal Vibration: Create the Life You Want with Law of Attraction Language, a min-e-book™

Are the words you speak bringing you closer to the life you want? Or are your word choices inadvertently creating more difficulties? Discover words and phrases that are part of the Language of Light in Absolute Love Publishing Creator Caroline A. Shearer's latest in the Raise Your Vibration min-e-book™ series: "Raise Your Verbal Vibration: Create the Life You Want with Law of Attraction Language." Learn what common phrases and words may be holding you back, and utilize a list of high-vibration words that you can begin to incorporate into your vocabulary. Increase your verbal vibration today with this compelling addition to the Raise Your Vibration series!

Raise Your Vibration: Tips and Tools for a High-Frequency Life, a min-e-book™

Presenting mind-opening concepts and tips, "Raise Your Vibration: Tips and Tools for a High-Frequency Life," a min-e-book™, opens the doorway to your highest and greatest good! This min-e-book™ demonstrates how every thought and every action affect our level of attraction, enabling us to attain what we truly want in life. Divided into categories of mind, body, and spirit/soul, readers will learn practical steps they can immediately put into practice to resonate at a higher vibration and further evolve their souls. A must-read primer for a higher existence! Are you ready for a high-frequency life?

The Weight Loss Shift: Be More, Weigh Less by Michelle Hastie

"The Weight Loss Shift: Be More, Weigh Less" by Michelle Hastie helps those searching for their ideal bodies shift into a higher way of being, inviting the lasting weight they want – along with the life of their dreams! Skip the diets and the gimmicks, "The Weight Loss Shift" is a permanent weight loss solution. Based on science, psychology, and spirituality, Hastie helps readers discover their ideal way of being through detailed instructions and exercises, and then helps readers transform to living a life free from worry about weight – forever!

Would you like to love your body at any weight? Would you like to filter through others' body expectations to discover your own? Would you like to live at your ideal weight naturally, effortlessly, and happily? Then, make the shift with "The Weight Loss Shift: Be More, Weigh Less!"

Where Is the Gift? Discovering the Blessing in Every Situation, a min-e-book™

Inside every challenge is a beautiful blessing waiting for us to unwrap it. All it takes is our choice to learn the lesson of the challenge! Are you in a situation that is challenging you? Are you struggling with finding the perfect blessing the universe is holding for you? This min-e-book™ will help you unwrap your blessings with more ease and grace, trust in the perfect manifestation of your life's challenges, and move through life with the smooth path your higher self intended. Make the choice: unwrap your gift today!

Women Will Save the World

Leading women across the nation celebrate the feminine nature through stories of collaboration, creativity, intuition, nurturing, strength, trailblazing, and wisdom in "Women Will Save the World." Inspired by a quote from the Dalai Lama, bestselling author and Absolute Love Publishing Founder Caroline A. Shearer brings these inherent feminine qualities to the forefront, inviting a discussion of the impact women have on humanity and initiating the question: Will Women Save the World?

All Books Available at
www.AbsoluteLovePublishing.com.

CPSIA information can be obtained
at www.ICGtesting.com
Printed in the USA
FSOW02n0917120217
30733FS